Methylene Blue

Dr Peter Baratosy MBBS FACNEM

Dr Peter Baratosy is a registered Medical Doctor in Australia. He obtained his medical degree from the University of Adelaide Medical School in 1978. He is a Fellow of the Australasian College of Nutritional and Environmental Medicine, and a member of the Australian and New Zealand College of Cannabis Prescribers. He is an accredited Medical Acupuncturist with the Medical Board of Australia.

Published by Dr Peter Baratosy 2026

Copyright Dr Peter Baratosy 2026

Cover Design Nikola Boskovski

Edited Karen Mace

Formatting Nikola Boskovski

ISBN 978-1-7637752-1-3 (print version)

978-1-7637752-2-0 (e Book)

Dedicated, as always, to my darling Jenny. Thank you for all your love, support and encouragement. I could not have achieved this without you.

I also dedicate this book to all those giants on whose shoulders I stand. To all the men and women who have done the research and without whom this book could not have been written.

Table of Contents

Books by the same author

CBD Oil: The Gift of Nature
ISBN 978-0-6451053-2-2

Hypothyroid Syndrome
ISBN 978-0-6451053-3-9

You and Your Gut
ISBN 978-0-6451053-5-3

Death by Civilization
ISBN 978-0-6451053-7-7

You and Your Hormones
ISBN 978-0-6451053-9-1

Books can be ordered through any bookshop or on-line.

FOREWORD

I have read Dr Peter Baratosy's methylene blue book and love it. I am grateful to Dr Baratosy for writing such a well-researched and referenced book.

I have been using methylene blue for a short time (18 months) and I have learned a lot through reading this book. I have been using it to treat Long Covid, MND, CFS and neuropathy, and was surprised to see that it has the potential for use in so many more illnesses.

The link to TCAs and MAOIs is fascinating reading as is the detail about the chemistry and history of methylene blue.

All who read the book will find very useful the tips on hormesis and dosing as well as the detailed, helpful information about contraindications and precautions.

The book is easy to read and, therefore, is as accessible to the average reader wanting to learn more about managing their own health, as it is to medical colleagues and other health professionals.

Dr Peter Baratosy MBBS FACNEM

Peter Baratosy's ability to communicate to us his interests, his research and his thoughts, is a gift.

Dr Sinclair Bode MBBS FACNEM

INTRODUCTION

I first came across methylene blue (MB) a few years ago when a colleague started treating a patient of mine. He had Parkinson's disease and unfortunately made little response with the medicinal cannabis that I had started. He consulted with my colleague, and later she told me that she had started him on MB. As I had not heard of this before, I asked her for more information. She gave me a pamphlet on MB, which I read through, put aside for further reference, then totally forgot about it.

Unfortunately, the patient has been lost to follow-up, so I do not know if there was any improvement.

Recently, I was reminded of MB by my wife. She is a great one for watching many YouTube videos and she mentioned that she saw an interesting video on MB. This reignited my interest in MB, and I looked around for the pamphlet, which I couldn't find! I asked my colleague for another copy and had a good read. At this same time, my wife ordered a bottle of MB online, with the view to experimenting on ourselves. While we were waiting for the bottle to arrive, I started reading and researching the topic which became increasingly interesting.

As I continued researching and learning more about MB, I realised, that like most things on the internet, there is a lot of information – as well as misinformation. So, I sifted through the good, the bad and the ugly!

There are many sites criticizing MB, saying it is a poison and can kill you. They claim it is nothing more than aquarium disinfectant! This is reminiscent of the ivermectin horse de-wormer saga. However, here I must point out that if you want to take MB, use pharmaceutical grade MB. Do not use aquarium disinfectant. While it does contain MB, there are also other substances that probably will not do you any good if swallowed.

Others have criticized MB, saying it is dangerous. To some extent this is true, though the same can be said for any drug, pharmaceutical, vitamin, herb, and nutrient. One of the most important factors is dosage. Another important factor is that it is contra-indicated in some people. So, yes – high doses can be dangerous. Giving it to certain people can be dangerous. It is the responsibility of the prescribing doctor to give the correct dose, to people who can take it without issue.

> *"Dosis sola facit venenum."*
> (translated *"Only the dose makes the poison"*)
> Theophrastus Bombastus Von Hohenheim
> (also known as Paracelsus (c1493 – 1541)

The threat of *serotonin syndrome* is always mentioned when discussing MB. This is almost used as a threat to scare people *not* to use it. I should point out here that nearly all case reports of serotonin syndrome caused by MB are based on MB given intravenously (IV) and in large doses in a hospital and/or surgical situation. It is probably not as dangerous as made out, especially with small regular oral doses. I could find only one case report where oral MB caused a serotonin syndrome; see Zuschlag, Warren, and Schultz, (2018).

Then there are sites which say MB is the best thing since sliced bread! Who is correct? Like many things, the truth is somewhere in between.

As I sifted through them, I found many sites that gave valuable information, but often the information was not referenced, and I need to see peer-reviewed references. For example, some sites discuss *"a study in 2023 showed that...."* but the actual reference was not detailed, or if there was a reference, when I tried to find it – many times it was wrong, or it didn't exist! That was very frustrating. I searched PubMed and found many journal papers written about MB, so I decided to gather these papers and to write a book about it.

There are some human, double-blind studies, but there aren't many big studies, mainly because studies are expensive. MB is off-patent and cheap, and so I doubt that any pharmaceutical company will spend a lot to study an off-patent and cheap product.

I have tried to collect the latest studies and present them to you, so that you can make an informed choice whether you want to try MB for your medical condition. While I encourage you to speak with your doctor, I am mindful that many doctors are not aware of the use of MB as a therapeutic medication. I suggest you find a doctor who understands MB.

WHAT IS METHYLENE BLUE?

Methylene Blue (MB) is also known as methylthi-oninium chloride. The International Union of Pure and Applied Chemistry standardised name is [3,7-bis(dime-thylamino) phenothiazine chloride tetra methylthionine chloride] (Khan et al., 2022).

Chemically it is a tricyclic phenothiazine.

The chemical formula is $C_{16}H_{18}N_3SCl$.

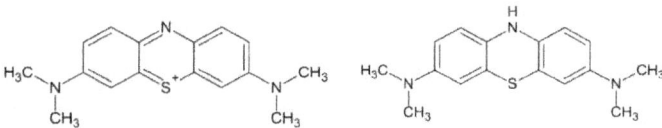

Methylene Blue   *LeucoMethylene Blue*

(Tucker, Lu, & Zhang, 2018)

This compound was first developed by a German scientist, Heinrich Cato in 1876 at the *Badische Anilin-und Sodafabrik* (German for 'Baden Aniline and Soda Factory' - BASF – this company is still around) and be-cause of its deep dark blue colour, it was first used as a textile dye. The original denim "blue jeans" manufactured in the late 1800s were dyed with MB.

The medical profession began to take notice. They found that MB could stain tissues and so it was used in pathology to stain and examine pathological specimens. Later it was discovered to have medicinal properties.

In 1886, Paul Ehrlich (1854 – 1915 Nobel-Prize winning German physician) noticed that MB turned *Plasmodium*, the parasite that causes malaria, blue. Since the malaria parasite would take up the blue dye, he concluded that MB might be used to selectively target malaria in the human body. Later, he used it to treat "swamp fever", another name for malaria, successfully. This was the first time that a synthetic substance was used to treat an infectious disease. Up to that point in time, quinine, extracted from the bark of the cinchona tree was the only treatment known (da Silva, Barreto de Abreu, Geraldes, & Nascimento, 2021).

The Spanish Jesuit missionaries in Peru learned about the medicinal properties of the bark of this tree from the local indigenous population. The local tribes used the bark to reduce fevers.

Here the legend and history diverge! Accounts vary.

Some accounts state that in 1630, Lady Ana de Osorio, the wife of the new Viceroy, Luis Xerónimo

Fernandes de Cabrera Bobadilla y Mendoza, 4th Count of Chinchón (1589-1647), went to Peru. Other accounts say the countess' name was Francisca Henriquez de Ribera (? – 1641). It turns out that she was the viceroy's second wife. His first wife was Ana de Osorio who is thought to have died in 1624. Though some sources say she died in 1639.

This lady (whichever was her name) was the Countess of Chinchón, the wife of the new Viceroy. Soon after arrival, she developed an illness with high fever thought to be malaria and almost died. The Jesuits recommended the use of this bark and so the story goes, saved the life of the countess. The story continues that in gratitude, she collected large amounts of bark and distributed it, partly in person and partly via the Jesuits, to those suffering from malaria.

Here history and legend diverge again!

She was supposed to have returned to Europe and spread the use of the tree bark throughout Spain and Europe, but she died in 1641 in Cartagena de Indus, present day Columbia, during her journey back to Spain. Other accounts suggest that it was the Viceroy himself who developed malaria and was saved by the cinchona bark.

It was probably the Jesuit missionary, Barnabé de Cobo (1582–1657) who introduced the bark to Europe, as the bark was known as Jesuits' bark. Other names include Contessa's powder, Peruvian bark or China bark. Cinchona bark contains many ingredients and the main component that has the antimalarial action is quinine. Before quinine, was isolated, the cinchona bark was pulverised into a fine powder and mixed into a liquid, generally wine, and then drunk.

"In 1820, quinine was extracted from the bark, isolated and named by Pierre Joseph Pelletier and Joseph Caventou. Purified quinine then replaced the bark as the standard treatment for malaria" (Achan et al., 2011).

It was not until 1944 that quinine was successfully synthesized by Robert Burns Woodward (1917-1989), the 1965 Nobel Prize winner in chemistry and William von Eggers Doering (1917-2011).

In England, the Lord Protector, Oliver Cromwell (1599–1658) was supposed to have died of malaria because he did not trust "Jesuits' bark" due to hatred of all things Catholic. He thought it was a "Papist poison" (Wood, 2015). However, by 1677, the Royal College of Physicians listed cinchona as the official malaria medicine.

An interesting fact is that the Cinchona tree grows high in the Andes mountains where there is no malaria. In one reference, the locals referred to the tree as *quinaquina* and that is where the name quinine comes from. Another interpretation is that in the local language, the bark of the tree was called *kina,* which the Spanish called *quina* – hence the name quinine. (https://unexaminedmedicine.org/2023/01/28/the-story-of-cinchona-from-myth-to-medi-cine/#:~:text=The%20story%20of%20the%20cin-chona,revolutionise%20the%20treat-ment%20of%20malaria. Accessed 13 March 2025).

While we are on the topic of quinine, the world-famous drink, the gin and tonic (G and T) was developed in India when the army of the East India Company was ordered to take quinine to protect them from malaria. The quinine drink was very unpleasant, so the officers added water, sugar, lime and gin to the quinine to make it more palatable – and so the G and T was born.

The countess's name was immortalised by Linnaeus (1707-1778), the Swedish biologist who formalised the naming of organisms, when he named the tree Cinchona, after her. However, due to a spelling mistake, it should have been Chinchona!

The legend and the truth about the discovery of cinchona bark treating malaria is complicated and much is still unknown and probably never will be known! However, this is not the main subject of the book. If you want to learn more about the above, see Miller, Rojas-Jaimes, Low, and Corbellini, (2022).

I have really gone off the topic!

Back to MB.

MB was used to treat malaria, but by the early 20th century, it was replaced by new synthetic antimalarials. The first antimalarial, pamaquine (also known as plasmochin) was derived from MB by German scientists in 1924. In 1926, German pharmacologist Wilhelm Roehl (1881-1929) proved it to be effective against malaria (Baird, 2019).

Pamaquine is no longer used due to its toxicity and there are more effective and less toxic antimalarial drugs in current use. The well-known antimalarial, chloroquine, was synthesized in 1934 by Hans Andersag (1902-1955). This was also derived from MB.

Hydroxychloroquine, which is chloroquine with an -OH group added was synthesized in the 1950s. It is very similar to chloroquine.

The early synthetic medicines were derived from the various dyes that had been discovered. At that time, the word dye and drug were almost interchangeable.

Some of the early antimalarials were derived from MB. The problem with dyes is that they stain - MB can stain people blue, and another compound, quinacrine, could stain people yellow; and it is not jaundice.

By 1995, due to the development of resistance to the current antimalarials, MB was again considered. MB was found to inhibit *glutathione reductase* in the malaria parasite, and it was also discovered that there were high levels of glutathione in the chloroquine (CQ) resistant strains. Clinical trials were started combining artemisinin-based combination therapy (ACT), with MB. *"MB was consistently shown to be highly effective in all endemic areas and demonstrated a strong effect on P. falciparum gametocyte reduction and synergy with ACT"* The researchers concluded that *"Adding MB to ACT could be a valuable approach for the prevention of resistance development and for transmission reduction in control and elimination programs"* (Lu et al., 2018).

The combination of chloroquine and MB has been trialled and found to be effective against chloroquine-resistant malaria. The researchers also showed that although the combination does reduce chloroquine bioavailability, it is not clinically relevant and is of minimal concern (Rengelshausen et al., 2004).

MB can work well as a monotherapy but does work more efficiently in combination. There is no evidence that malaria can develop a resistance to MB (Lu et al., 2018).

Unfortunately, MB use fell into oblivion as newer, synthetic drugs were discovered and became the preferred anti-malarial treatment. MB was used during World War 1 (WW1) by Germany because of the inability to source cinchona bark which was then the current treatment for malaria.

During World War 2 (WW2), malaria was a huge problem in the Southwest Pacific theatre. The commander of the allied forces, General Douglas McArthur stated, *"This will be a long war, if for every division I have facing the enemy, I must count on a second division in the hospital with malaria, and a third division convalescing from this debilitating disease"* (Schirmer, Adler, Pickhardt, & Mandelkow, 2011).

MB was used during WW2 but was disliked by the soldiers due to the development of blue urine.

During the Vietnam war, as malaria started to become resistant to the drugs used, MB use was re-considered. Studies did show it was effective especially in conjunction with other dugs but there was poor compliance due to the development of blue sclera and blue urine, as well as the gastrointestinal side effects. This was probably due to the large doses that were needed. One veteran recalled that they had to take the dose as *"teaspoons of the MB crystals."*

There has been a resurgence in the use of MB to treat malaria.

In 2010, Boutogo et al. concluded that *"MB acts slowly against the blood stages of P. falciparum. MB alone needs to be given for at least 7 days to be efficacious in the treatment of falciparum malaria but should be used in combination with a fast acting antimalarial."*

The gametocyte is that stage of the malaria parasite that the mosquito picks up when biting an infected person, which then can be spread to the next person. Conventional malaria treatment can kill off the parasite stage that causes the symptoms, but as the parasite is dying, it releases the gametocyte which can infect the mosquito and therefore spreads the disease. MB has been shown to kill the gametocyte.

Coulibaly et al. (2009) studied 180 children between ages 6-10 in Burkina Faso with uncomplicated falciparum malaria, who were randomised to 1) MB-artesunate (AS), 2) MB-amodiaquine (AQ), and 3) AS-AQ (local standard of care). Both MB-containing regimens were associated with significantly reduced gametocyte carrier rates during follow-up days 3, 7, and 14.

MB was also noted to have antimicrobial properties and was used to treat wounds and infections and as a disinfectant in surgery. Prior to the discovery of penicillin, MB was used to treat wounded soldiers during World War 1. In the beginning of the twentieth century, MB was used for many medical and hygienic practices.

MB was found to be particularly useful in psychiatry. Initially it was added to psychiatric medication, mostly to monitor compliance! The MB turned the patient's urine blue, so the doctors could see if patients were taking their medication. Later, it was discovered that MB itself had antidepressant and other positive psychotropic properties. Further research used MB as the parent molecule in the development of chlorpromazine and the tricyclic antidepressants. Note that chemically, MB is a tricyclic phenothiazine compound.

MB was also used to test compliance during the dexamethasone suppression test (DST). Kraus et al. (1987) showed that adding MB to dexamethasone was found to readily validate compliance and did not influence the DST results.

Before I go any further, one important aspect should be mentioned. MB is not necessarily a standalone treatment. MB should be part of a wholistic approach; used in conjunction with other actions such as diet, exercise, nutrient supplements, herbs, lifestyle, adequate sleep, sunshine, stress reduction, and so on. These all join to help the body achieve an overall better health and improve the quality of life.

CURRENT USE OF METHYLENE BLUE

MB is still being used today.

As a pathology stain

MB can be very useful in the pathology laboratory, staining tissue samples and examining them under the microscope.

- MB is used to determine cell viability. MB will turn clear (leucoMB) with healthy cells and stay blue with dead or damaged cells.
- MB can be used to stain bacteria to aid identification. It is different from the Gram staining method (named after the Danish bacteriologist Hans Christian Gram (1853-1938), dividing bacteria into Gram-positive, and Gram-negative bacteria. MB is a quick method to highlight bacteria in specimens.
- MB can be used to identify nucleic acids – RNA and DNA.

- MB can be used to identify cellular structures.
- MB can be used to identify between bacterial, viral and fungal diseases.
- MB is a positively charged molecule and therefore attracted to negatively charged molecules such as RNA, DNA, and polyphosphates.

Methaemoglobinaemia

MB is used currently in the treatment of methaemoglobinaemia. Methaemoglobinaemia is a condition where the blood cannot carry oxygen. The basic underlying problem is that the iron in the haemoglobin molecule is changed from the ferrous (Fe^{++}) to the ferric (Fe^{+++}) form. This prevents the molecule from picking up oxygen and carrying it around the body. The symptoms are related to oxygen deficiency – which include headache, dizziness, shortness of breath, tachycardia, fatigue/lethargy, nausea, confusion, loss of consciousness, and blue-coloured skin. Causes include certain medication, foods, chemicals, or it can be inherited. The substances include benzocaine and other local anaesthetics, nitrites, antimalarials and dapsone. Foods that contain nitrites (includes beets, carrots, green beans, spinach, squash) may also be a cause, especially in children. Paradoxically, high doses of MB can cause methaemoglobinaemia! This is an example of the hermetic effect, which will be discussed later.

Note that in normal people there is generally a small amount of methaemoglobin, generally less than 1%.

The "blue people" of Kentucky

The Fugate family live in the hills of Kentucky. They and related cousins, the Combs, Smiths, Ritchies and Stacys, have a congenital abnormality. They are known as the "blue people of Kentucky". They are quite literally blue due to a congenital form of methaemoglobinaemia. Due to the remoteness, and due to their blue colouring, they have been isolated from society and largely left to themselves. There has been significant inbreeding. As this genetic condition is caused by a recessive gene, with inbreeding, there are many in the family that have this condition. They can be literally "Smurf blue"!

The people with congenital methaemoglobinaemia generally have a methaemoglobin of between 10 to 20 percent. This amount gives the blue skin but generally none of the other issues. Many have had long healthy lives. Major symptoms only develop when the methaemoglobinaemia exceeds twenty percent.

In the early 1960s, some of the family members sought help from a haematologist from the University of Kentucky, Dr Madison Cawein (1925-1985). He studied them and discovered that they were suffering from congenital/genetic methaemoglobinaemia. He started treating them with MB, which converted the methaemoglobin back to functional normal haemoglobin.

Initially, MB was given intravenously. It is ironic that this bright blue dye removed the blue colouring and converted their skin to a normal pink colour. Initially many were sceptical when they saw the bright blue intravenous drip – a bright blue substance to fix their blue colouration, but in the end, they saw the benefits. A report of this was published in the *Archives of Internal Medicine*, Cawein, Behlen, Lappat, and Cohn, (1964).

As the condition was congenital, due to an absence of a critical enzyme *cytochrome-b5 methemoglobin reductase*, treatment must be continuous. Treatment was continued with regular oral MB capsules.

Treatment of methaemoglobinaemia today involves oxygen therapy, but if that is inadequate, MB can be administered intravenously at a rate of 1-2 mgs/kg over five minutes. A second dose may be given after 30-60 minutes if needed. Hyperbaric oxygen can also be used if it is available.

Carbon monoxide poisoning

MB can be used to treat carbon monoxide (CO) poisoning, though is not used as much today. Oxygen therapy and if available, hyperbaric oxygen therapy, is the mainstay of CO poisoning. In the past, however, MB was used as treatment for CO poisoning (Geiger, 1933).

One of the complications of acute CO poisoning is *delayed encephalopathy after carbon monoxide poisoning* (DEACMP). This is thought to be due to delayed cerebral damage related to oxidative stress. MB may be a promising agent to use after CO poisoning to prevent the delayed cerebral damage. Note that this study was done in a rat model (Zhao et al., 2018).

Cyanide poisoning

MB was used in the treatment of cyanide (CN) poisoning. Hanzlik (1933) wrote that Sahlin in 1926 demonstrated that MB was antidotal to cyanide. The use was significantly established by 1930 (Hanzik, 1933).

Treatment involves maintaining airways, decontamination (note that mouth-to-mouth is not recommended because of the risk of cyanide poisoning to the resuscitator) and oxygen therapy.

Hydroxocobalamin is the treatment of choice, given intravenously at a dose of 5 grams over 15 minutes. Other substances include sodium nitrite and sodium thiosulfate.

In 2018 Haouzi et al. revisited the use of MB in cyanide poisoning and following further research by the same researchers in 2020 they concluded that *"... MB mitigates the neuronal toxicity of CN in a dose-dependent manner, preventing the lethal depression of respiratory medullary neurons and fatal outcome."*

Ifosfamide-induced encephalopathy

Ifosfamide is a chemotherapeutic drug used on its own or with other agents in the treatment of various types of cancer. As with all chemotherapy, there are always side effects.

Ifosfamide has a particularly severe effect on the central nervous system (CNS) causing an encephalopathy in approximately 27% of cases that are treated (Sunela & Bärlund, 2016).

Pelgrims et al. (2000) showed that MB is an effective treatment for ifosfamide-induced encephalopathy. The researchers also suggested that MB can be used prophylactically.

Turner, Duong, and Good (2003) showed that in the acute situation, i.e. after ifosfamide treatment, CNS improvement occurred within 24 hours of MB administration. In the prophylactic situation, MB decreased the severity of symptoms significantly as compared to previous treatment cycles. This allowed patients to continue with ifosfamide therapy.

Abahssain et al. (2021) concluded that *"Methylene blue can be used as a treatment for IIE (*Ifosfamide-induced encephalopathy) *owing to the severity of the IIE as well as absence of standard medication."*

Vasoplegic syndrome/ Vasoplegic shock

Vasoplegia is a syndrome characterised by excessive low blood pressure due to reduced vascular resistance, yet with a normal cardiac output. This syndrome can develop in relation to septic shock, post cardiac bypass, and after surgery, burns and trauma (Lambden, Creagh-Brown, Hunt, Summers, & Forni, 2018).

MB has been used to treat vasoplegic shock after cardiac surgery. Levin et al. (2004) concluded that *"The use of methylene blue reduced the high mortality in this population."*

In a single-centre randomised controlled trial, Ibarra-Estrada et al. (2023) showed that the use of MB in septic shock reduced the stay in ICU and hospital without adverse effects.

Note that these above conditions are serious and can be life-threatening. Here the MB must be given intravenously and in high doses, in a hospital setting.

MB in surgical practice

MB is used in surgery as a diagnostic tool. Due to the bright blue colour, MB can also be used primarily as a dye to highlight structures, fistulae, etc. to make surgery safer.

Precise surgical debridement is essential to achieve effective wound closure. MB is applied topically to the wound, then wiped off. It is removed from normal tissue, but stains eschar, non-viable tissue and granulation tissue. This stained tissue is then surgically removed which makes wound closure better and safer for proper healing (Dorafshar, Gitman, Henry, Agarwal, & Gottlieb, 2010).

MB has also been used in parathyroid surgery. An intravenous infusion can highlight the diseased parathyroid glands which therefore make surgery safer and easier (Bewick & Pfleiderer, 2014).

Another use of MB is in breast cancer. MB can be injected near to the tumour to identify the first lymph node (sentinel) that drains the cancerous area. This helps in identifying and mapping of the sentinel nodes

(Zakaria, Hoskin, & Degnim, 2008). Surgeons then can more accurately remove the sentinel nodes.

A 2014 study showed that the accuracy rate was 93% with a false negative rate of 15% (Özdemir, Mayir, Demirbakan, & Oygür, 2014).

However, in a 2018 study, mapping sentinel node locations with MB alone had an acceptable identification rate, but an excessive false negative rate according to the American Society of Breast Surgeons' recommendations (Li, Chen, Qi, & Li, 2018).

Zou et al. (2019) also published a study where MB injections were used to highlight lymph nodes when performing axillary lymph node dissection.

Newer techniques, including CAT scanning with newer dyes or radioactive tracers are now being used (Goyal, 2018).

A similar technique can be used in the treatment of colorectal cancer. The decision whether adjuvant chemotherapy is required is based on histological lymph node evaluation.

Carvalho, Gonçalves, Teixeira, Goulart, and Leão (2024) analysed 18 trials looking at the use of intravenous MB in patients with colorectal cancer.

The study showed that *"The results of the statistical analysis of the lymph node harvest variable demonstrate a significant statistical difference between the group that received methylene blue injection and the group that underwent conventional dissection."*

What this means is that MB showed up more lymph nodes than can be generally detected just by conventional dissection.

MB can also be used as a tracer dye to discover fistulae (a fistula is a permanent abnormal passageway, usually permanent, between two organs in the body or between an organ and the exterior of the body), such as bronchopleural fistulae (Nasin et al., 2017), enterocutaneous fistulae (Botros et al., 2017), colonic fistulae (Ng Ying Kin, Wei, Arachchi, & Bolshinsky, 2021) and complex urinary fistulae (Hanash, Al Zahrani, Mokhtar, & Aslam, 2003).

Here the blue dye is injected into the fistula, which can help the surgeon to determine the course of the fistula.

Zhang, Liao, Ai, and Liu (2015) used MB to identify intersegmental planes in the lungs, so that segments with small tumours can be safely and accurately removed.

Adhesions can develop after abdominal surgery which can cause complications later. Seo, Choi, Lee, and Kang (2022) looked at MB for reduction of adhesions. The researchers performed a systematic review and meta-analysis of post abdominal surgery in a rat model. The researchers concluded that *"MB had a beneficial effect on intraperitoneal adhesion following laparotomy, and adhesions decreased with increase in dose."*

Neagoe, Ionica, and Mazilu (2018) used MB in patients with adhesions from previous abdominal surgery. These patients had further surgery to treat the adhesions. They concluded that *"The use of methylene blue during adhesiolysis surgery appears to reduce the recurrence of adhesion-related symptoms, suggesting a beneficial effect in the prevention of adhesion formation."*

MB has local anaesthetic properties.

Deng et al. (2025) injected an MB containing cocktail around the knee after arthroplasty. They concluded that *"Methylene blue combined with a cocktail can be safely used for local infiltration after knee arthroplasty, which reduces postoperative opioid consumption and suppresses the release of inflammatory factors. Moreover, it synergistically enhanced the local anesthetic analgesia and provided sustained pain relief for at least 4 weeks."*

Zhang et al. (2025) used MB injections after costal cartilage harvest. Pain can be quite significant post-surgery, and the study compared MB with ropivacaine (a local anaesthetic). The results showed that *"Patients receiving MB exhibited a significant decrease in pain scores from 5 days to 1 month of treatment compared to the ropivacaine group."*

Perianal surgery can be quite painful post operatively. Many have been known to postpone or even avoid surgery because of the anticipated post-operative pain with the consequence of the condition becoming much worse. Shareef et al. (2024) used MB injection after perianal surgery and concluded that *"The reduction in inflammation and nerve excitability, along with denervation, contribute to the analgesic effect and pain reduction of Methylene Blue."*

Azhough, Jalali, Dashti, Taher, and Aghajani (2024) studied 97 patients undergoing haemorrhoidectomy. A double-blind, randomised controlled trial compared intradermal injection of 1% MB with 0.5% Marcaine (local anaesthetic) injection as the control group. The study demonstrated *"... comparable efficacy in reducing post-hemorrhoidectomy pain, with negligible side effects and complications."*

In a systematic review and meta-analysis on the effect of local infiltration of methylene blue on post-hemorrhoidectomy pain, Wickramasinghe, Wickramasinghe, Samarasekera, and Warusavitarne (2025) concluded that *"This meta-analysis demonstrates that posthemorrhoidectomy pain is significantly lower in patients with MB infiltration, requiring less oral analgesia, and the infiltration of MB does not affect anal continence. The analgesic action seems to wear off between 7 and 14 days.*"

MB has been used in the treatment of pilonidal sinus. MB is carefully injected into the sinus, before surgery. The recurrence rate was reduced for two possible reasons.

1. The MB showed up the extent of the sinus, and a wider excision was performed because the blue dye showed the extent of the sinus tract. On the negative side, a larger area needs to be removed, which can initially produce more post-surgery complications, however, despite this, better outcomes were achieved as more of the sinus tract was removed.
2. MB has an antimicrobial effect (Durgut, 2018).

Doll et al. (2008) report that MB in pilonidal surgery reduces by half the long-term recurrence rates in acute pilonidal sinus disease.

The use of MB to detect abnormal cells during endoscopic biopsy in Barrett's oesophagitis has been shown to be more accurate than just random biopsies (Canto et al., 2000).

In contrast, Ragunath, Krasner, Raman, Haqqani, and Cheung (2003) showed that MB staining was superior to random biopsy for detecting specialised intestinal metaplasia, but not for detecting dysplasia or carcinoma. The researchers further state that although the staining technique prolongs the endoscopy slightly, it is a well-tolerated procedure.

These above uses are for in-hospital treatment for life-death situations, or during surgery. However, MB can be used for in-clinic treatments as well.

MB USES IN NON-HOSPITAL CLINICAL PRACTICE

The above uses for MB are in hospital situations and generally given in high doses by intravenous administration or injected into tissue during operative procedures.

What about non-hospital use?

The next section will discuss MB use in a low-dose, long-term oral administration. Of course, some of these uses are still being investigated and many of the studies have been done on animal models. On the other hand, we have seen that MB is safe when used appropriately. There is therefore no reason to wait for years before double-blind studies are done, as they may never be done since MB is off-patent and inexpensive.

As an antibiotic

MB has been used as an antibiotic. In the USA, but not in Australia, there is a MB product available over the counter (OTC) for urinary tract infections (UTI). The product treated the pain, discomfort, and frequency. This product contained MB 10.8 mgs, methenamine 81.6 mgs, benzoic acid 9.0 mgs, phenyl salicylate 36.2 mgs and hyoscyamine sulphate 0.12 mgs. There are many websites on the internet where women tell their story of how well this product works, not just for UTI but for interstitial cystitis and painful bladder syndrome.

In one study, Gama et al. (2020) compared *"... 2 urinary antiseptic combinations in the symptomatic treatment of recurrent cystitis: methenamine 120mg + methylene blue 20mg (Group A) versus acriflavine 15mg + methenamine 250mg + methylene blue 20mg + Atropa belladonna L. 15mg (Group B)."* The conclusion was that both treatments were effective in reducing UTI symptoms after 3 days. The methenamine + MB combination (group A) resulted in fewer treatment-related adverse effects.

Painful bladder syndrome (PBS) and a subgroup known as interstitial cystitis (IC) is a painful condition of the bladder occurring more frequently in women (90%). Symptoms include pain, frequency of urination and urgency. It can occur day and night. The filling of the bladder produces pain, and emptying the bladder can relieve some of the pain. This drives the frequent urination. Initially the condition can present as "flares", resembling a UTI (this therefore must be excluded). As the condition progresses, the symptoms become more constant. The cause is not known and there is no cure but there are some treatments. (https://aua.com.au/conditions-and-services/female-urology/interstitial-cystitis/ accessed 15 February 2025).

As mentioned earlier, there are many stories of women who have this condition and gain relief with the above product. However, while researching, I could not find any peer-reviewed references for the use of MB treating IC. As we shall see, MB has many properties including local anaesthetic effects and is an anti-inflammatory.

Oral MB turns the urine blue, therefore there must be MB in the urine, and it is in constant contact with the bladder wall, which should reduce inflammation and pain. In theory, therefore, MB *should* help IC. There is a need for studies to be done on this, as IC treatment is difficult at the best of times.

Intravesical MB has been suggested for IC but note that the bladder mucosa can be quite sensitive and large doses of MB instilled into the bladder may cause aggravation. Oral MB ends up in the bladder at lower doses and may improve the condition without causing aggravation.

One of the treatments for IC is a drug called amitriptyline, a tricyclic antidepressant. It is ironic that the tricyclic antidepressants were developed originally from MB!

Birder (2019) wrote *"In addition, interstitial cystitis/bladder pain syndrome symptoms can frequently overlap with other conditions including <u>irritable bowel syndrome, fibromyalgia, chronic fatigue syndrome, anxiety disorders, and a number of other syndromes not directly related to the urinary bladder.</u>"* (emphasis the author)

Since MB is known to influence some of those conditions, i.e. fibromyalgia, chronic fatigue, anxiety, and so on, it could be helpful in the wholistic treatment of this condition as well.

Treat the patient with symptoms, not necessarily the name of the condition.

Anti-viral activity

MB can also act as an antiviral.

Cagno et al. (2021) used MB against the H1N1 influenza virus and SARS-CoV-2 virus. This was an *in vitro* study of cells infected with these viruses and showed that MB displayed virucidal preventative and therapeutic activity.

Similar conclusions were reached by Dabholkar et al. (2021) and Gendrot et al. (2020).

"Based on studies, MB can simultaneously affect most of the host's harmful responses caused by SARS-CoV-2 infection due to its multiple properties, including anti-hypoxemia, anti-oxidant, [sic] immune system modulator, and antiviral" (Emadi, Hamidi Alamdari, Attaran, & Attaran, 2024).

Li et al. (2020) showed MB is a potent and broad-spectrum inhibitor of Zika virus and Dengue virus.

Chronic conditions

Research has shown that MB can be used to treat a multitude of conditions. This is because of its effect on the mitochondria. Mitochondria are the intracellular organelles that have been described as the *"powerhouse of the cell."* The mitochondria require an exchange of electrons to produce adenosine triphosphate (ATP), the energy molecule of the cell. This is achieved via the electron transport chain (ETC).

MB is a tricyclic phenothiazine molecule and is a blue colour but when it undergoes a redox cycle, MB is reduced by nicotinamide adenine dinucleotide phosphate (NADPH) to make leucoMB, an uncharged clear compound. LeucoMB is then re-oxidised by oxygen back to

MB. This cyclic redox process is continuous. As an anti-oxidant, MB reduces oxidative stress, which is an imbalance between free radicals and antioxidant activity. This reduces cellular damage which can contribute to ageing and various diseases. The bottom line is that MB acts as an electron donor and an electron acceptor.

Oxidised MB is an electron acceptor; this is in its blue colour state. In this form it can participate in mitochondrial function in the ETC, as well as contribute to removal of free radicals, by accepting electrons from free radicals, thus protecting the cells from oxidative damage.

Reduced MB, also known as leucoMB, which is a clear state, is an electron donor. This aids detoxification and protects cells from oxidative damage.

MB is excreted in the urine as a mixture of MB, leucoMB, and demethylated metabolites such as azure A and azure B. This is the reason for the blue/green urine colour; it looks unusual but is harmless. People need to be warned, as it could frighten some.

The ETC is a series of electron transporters in the inner mitochondrial membrane, and its purpose is to shuttle electrons from NADH to FADH2 to oxygen.

The ETC is comprised of five complexes:

Complex 1 - NADH-ubiquinone oxidoreductase.

Complex 2 - succinate dehydrogenase.

These are the entrances for electrons where NADH and FADH2 transfers electrons to Complex 1 and 2.

These electrons are transported by –

Complex 3 - CoQ-cytochrome c reductase, and

Complex 4 – cytochrome c oxidase.

With the help of co-enzyme Q10 (CoQ10), Complex 3 transfers electrons to cytochrome c and Complex 4 transfers electrons from cytochrome c to oxygen to generate H2O. In this process, Complex 5 – ATP synthase generates ATP by phosphorylating ADP (Xue, Thaivalappil, & Cao, 2021).

Reactive oxygen species (ROS) is a main byproduct of this process – there are 11 sites of ROS generation, and most are in Complex 1.

Mitochondrial dysfunction leads to oxidative damage, primarily damaging Complexes 1 and 5.

MB is hydrophilic and lipophilic which means that it is highly permeable through membranes. It is also positively charged. MB can readily cycle between the oxidised and reduced forms, and this characteristic allows it to be a catalytic redox cycler in mitochondria, promoting cytochrome oxidase activity and ATP production. MB also reduces ROS production by bypassing Complex 1/3 activity.

"MB receives electrons from NADH through Complex I, converting to leucoMB. LeucoMB can directly transfer these electrons to cytochrome c, re-oxidized to MB. Therefore, MB has the potential to protect cells against oxidative stress under pathological conditions" (Xue, Thaivalappil, & Cao, 2021).

MB, in the past, has been shown to photo-inactivate bacteria, is a potent antiviral and is also an antifungal and anti-parasitic. These are the reasons that MB is used in aquariums as a disinfectant.

MB also is used in photodynamic therapy in cancer, including lung cancer, breast, and prostate cancer.

Photodynamic therapy

"Photodynamic therapy (PDT) is a minimally invasive therapeutic modality that has gained great attention in the past years as a new therapy for cancer treatment" (Correia, Rodrigues, Pimenta, Dong, & Yang, 2021).

The technique uses photosensitisers that react with light to form reactive oxygen species in the target tissues, resulting in cellular death.

One such photosensitiser is MB, which has an absorption spectrum in the 550-700nm region. This is the near infrared and red region.

Light activates MB and transitions it to an excited state which allows it to generate reactive oxygen species (ROS) which is essential for its antibacterial, antiviral, antifungal and anticancer properties.

This can be useful in many situations, including chronic infections, viral lesions such as warts and molluscum contagiosum, and chronic nasal infections such as Staphylococcus biofilms, rhinosinusitis, antibiotic resistant bacteria and so on (Kaura et al., 2020).

Taldaev et al. (2023) concluded that *"The results of the systematic review support the suggestions that photodynamic therapy with methylene blue helps against different types of cancer, including colorectal tumor, carcinoma, and melanoma."*

The light source can be xenon lamps, light emitting diodes (LED), laser beams or fibre optic devices. The popularity of the red LED therapy has increased, and these devices are relatively inexpensive. One simple source of light is sunlight. This has many wavelengths and causes shallow skin penetration, however, there is difficulty accurately controlling the dose (Polat & Kang, 2021).

On the other hand, sitting in the sun can be therapeutic, is easy to achieve and is free! As an added bonus, vitamin D is produced by the action of sunlight on the skin.

Remember - sun exposure not sunburn!

Mitochondrial dysfunction

Mitochondrial disease/dysfunction, as the name suggests, is a condition that affects the workings of the mitochondria. The purpose of mitochondria is to produce energy for the cells and therefore for the whole body. Every cell in the body contains mitochondria, but some tissues have more than others – specifically the brain, heart and muscles. From this we can conclude that if there is mitochondrial dysfunction then it is the brain, heart and muscles that bear the brunt. Again, we can conclude that the symptoms would include brain dysfunction, weakness and tiredness.

There are basically two types of mitochondrial dysfunction: primary mitochondrial dysfunction (PMD) and secondary mitochondrial dysfunction (SMD).

Primary mitochondrial dysfunction (PMD)

PMD is largely genetic and therefore congenital. *"Pmds can occur due to germline mutations in mitochondrial DNA (mtDNA) and/or nuclear DNA (nDNA) genes encoding ETC proteins"* (Niyazov, Kahler, & Frye, 2016).

The symptoms do vary, as does onset and severity and can be mild to critical. Examples include Alper's disease, mitochondrial myopathy, maternally inherited diabetes mellitus and deafness (MIDD), Kearns-Sayre syndrome, Pearson syndrome, Leber's hereditary optic neuropathy (LHON), Leigh syndrome and many others. With the improvement in gene abnormality detecting technology, new diseases are continually being discovered.

The incidence is relatively rare; about 1 in 4,000 children in the USA will develop mitochondrial disease by the age of 10.

Secondary mitochondrial dysfunction (SMD)

"Secondary mitochondrial dysfunction (SMD) can be caused by genes encoding neither function nor production of the oxphos proteins and accompanies many hereditary non-mitochondrial diseases. SMD may also be due to nongenetic causes such as environmental

factors." The researchers continued *"... SMD commonly accompanies many non-PMD disorders, supporting evidence that SMD is likely much more common than PMD"* (Niyazov, Kahler, & Frye, 2016).

This can also be referred to as acquired mitochondrial dysfunction. There are many conditions that have secondary (acquired) mitochondrial dysfunction. These include:

- Amyotrophic lateral sclerosis (ALS).
- Alzheimer's disease.
- Neuropsychiatric disorders; bipolar disorder, schizophrenia, anxiety, depression.
- Ageing and senescence.
- Cancer.
- Metabolic syndrome, including diabetes, hypertension, cardiovascular disease.
- Neurodegenerative diseases - Huntington's disease, Parkinson's disease, multiple sclerosis.
- Long COVID.
- Chronic fatigue syndrome (CFS), myalgic encephalomyelitis (ME).
- Autism/ADHD.
- Post-concussion syndrome.
- Sarcopoenia.
- Other miscellaneous issues.

The SMD may not necessarily be a *cause* of the disease/condition but is associated with it and treating the mitochondrial dysfunction can possibly help improve the condition.

MB as anti-inflammatory

MB has been shown to have anti-inflammatory properties. Li and Ying (2023) showed in a mouse model that MB reduced the level of interleukin-6 (IL-6), as well as other actions which reduce inflammation. The researchers concluded that MB has therapeutic potential for multiple inflammation-associated diseases.

Inflammasomes are multi-protein complexes that mature interleukins which are related to inflammation. Ahn et al. (2017) showed that MB attenuated inflammasome activation.

Rats were given sodium hydroxide to induce oesophageal burns. MB was shown to reduce inflammation and prevent the formation of scarring and stenoses. The researchers concluded that *"MB is effective in treating tissue damage caused by corrosive esophageal burns and in preventing esophageal stenosis. Complication rates of corrosive esophageal burns may be decreased by using MB in the initial treatment stage"* (Şen Tanrıkulu et al., 2019).

Li et al. (2022) showed in a rat osteoarthritis model that MB injected into the joint protected cartilage, reduced synovitis and reduced pain. This shows the MB anti-inflammatory activity.

Zheng and Li (2019) showed MB inhibits the inflammatory response by targeting the mechanism that regulates inflammation.

MB has anti-inflammatory action, therefore can be useful in most situations as inflammation is the basis of many diseases.

> Inflammation is the basis of many diseases.

Amyotrophic lateral sclerosis (ALS)

Amyotrophic lateral sclerosis (ALS), often called Lou Gehrig's disease (Lou Gehrig - American baseball player 1903–1941) is a neurodegenerative disease involving the nerve cells in the brain and spinal cord that causes loss of muscle control. The condition generally starts with twitching and weakness in an arm or leg, difficulty swallowing or slurred speech. Eventually all muscles are affected and there is difficulty with moving, eating, speaking and breathing. There is no cure.

"Mitochondrial dysfunction is a prevalent feature of many neurodegenerative diseases including motor neuron disorders such as <u>amyotrophic lateral sclerosis (ALS)</u>." (Emphasis the author). The authors continue *"Disruption of mitochondrial structure, dynamics, bioenergetics and calcium buffering has been extensively reported in ALS patients and model systems and has been suggested to be directly involved in disease pathogenesis"* (Smith, Shaw, & De Vos, 2019).

The role of MB in mitochondrial dysfunction has produced much interest recently. As we have already seen, MB can reroute electrons in the ETC, increasing activity in Complex 4 and promoting mitochondrial activity while also dealing with oxidative stress. Tucker, Lu, and Zhang (2018) state that *"... MB has shown impressive efficacy in mitigating neurodegeneration and the accompanying behavioral phenotypes in animal models for such conditions as stroke, global cerebral ischemia, Alzheimer's disease, Parkinson's disease, and traumatic brain injury."* This study refers to the action of MB in animal studies. Can this be translated to humans?

Possibly.

However, in one study in a mouse model of ALS, Audet, Soucy, and Julien (2012) showed that despite MB having established neuroprotective properties, MB failed to protect in a mouse model of ALS.

As noted above, there is no treatment for ALS, and since MB is a very safe compound, there is no reason not to use it in this condition.

Alzheimer's disease (AD)

Alzheimer's disease (AD) is a neurodegenerative disease that generally starts after the age of 65, though there is a "young onset Alzheimer's disease" that starts before the age of 65. This is a cause of 60-70% of dementia cases. Memory loss (that disrupts daily life) of recent events is one of the first early symptom, which slowly progresses. As the disease advances, problems with language, disorientation, mood swings, loss of motivation, self-neglect and behaviour issues develop. Gradually there is withdrawal from family and society, and further deterioration leads to loss of bodily functions and ultimately death. There is no cure.

I have discussed AD in my previous books in relation to metabolic syndrome (**Death by Civilization**) and in relation to hormones (**You and Your Hormones**).

However, we can look at AD from a deeper level.

AD is a neurodegenerative disease and as noted above, Tucker, Lu, and Zhang (2018) consider mitochondrial dysfunction as an underlying cause.

McGill-Percy, Liu, and Qi (2025) came to the same conclusion.

Here again, MB can be considered as a treatment for AD, as MB enhances the action of mitochondria.

Medina, Caccamo, and Oddo (2011) made comment on a phase 2 study where MB showed improvements in AD patients after six months treatment. To explain how MB acts on the brain, the researchers used a mouse model (3xTg-AD) where the mouse develops age dependant accumulation of amyloid beta (Aβ) and tau. Aβ and tau are proteins that build up into plaques and tangles which damage the neurons and cause the memory and cognitive decline in AD. The researchers showed that MB reduces Aβ levels and improves learning and cognitive decline.

Hashmi et al. (2023) published a comprehensive review of randomised control trials. They concluded that *"The literature review includes randomized clinical trials investigating MB's potential benefits in treating AD. The findings of the studies indicate that the administration of MB has demonstrated enhancements in cognitive function, reductions in the accumulation of plaques containing beta-amyloid, improvements in memory and cognitive function in animal subjects, and possesses antioxidant properties that can mitigate oxidative stress and inflammation within the brain."*

Rodriguez et al. (2016) showed that a single low dose of MB can *"increase functional MR imaging activity during sustained attention and short-term memory tasks and enhance memory retrieval."* This was measured using functional MRI imaging.

If MB can do this to a normal brain, it could possibly help with AD. As noted earlier, there is no specific treatment for AD. Much of the current research is with animal models, however, there is no reason NOT to try MB in AD. Any treatment that may help should be used, especially if that treatment has an excellent safety profile.

Case study 1

A 40-year-old lady presented with a strong family history of Alzheimer's disease (AD). She was obviously concerned that she may develop this disease. Tests, including brain scans showed no evidence of any brain abnormality. However, her APO E genotype showed she had an APO E 4 gene which is associated with AD. I started her on MB. She later told me that she advised all her family members to start MB. Will this prevent or modify AD? We may not know for many years, but it is better than doing nothing and hoping. The treatment is simple and safe and has scientific backing.

Neuropsychiatric disorders

As noted earlier, MB was used in psychiatric practice over a century ago. It was the first synthetic drug
ever used to treat pain, malaria and psychotic disorders.
Chlorpromazine, discovered in 1951, by Paul Charpentier, in the laboratories of Rhône-Poulenc, a French pharmaceutical company, is regarded as the first synthetic an-
tipsychotic drug. However, it is important to point out
that MB was used at least 50 years earlier, and it is also
important to point out that chlorpromazine was derived
from MB. MB was used to treat psychotic patients, and
bipolar and unipolar patients (Howland, 2016).

*"This drug [MB] also inhibits the activity of mon-
oamine oxidase, nitric oxide synthase, and guanylyl
cyclase, as well as tau protein aggregation; increases the
release of neurotransmitters, such as serotonin and norepinephrine; reduces amyloid-beta levels; and increases
cholinergic transmission"* (Howland, 2016).

These properties make MB useful for psychotic illnesses, depression, AD, and a host of other neurodegenerative diseases.

Just as a minor deviation, another drug that is still
in use, and was derived from MB is promethazine, the
antihistamine. Paul Charpentier, a scientist working at
Rhône Poulenc (later Sanofi-Aventis) developed this
drug in the 1940s. One side effect is drowsiness. With

the development of non-sedating antihistamines, promethazine is used more for the drowsiness side effect to help sleep, rather than as an antihistamine.

MB is a mono amine oxidase (MAO) inhibiter. MAO is an enzyme that breaks down serotonin. Therefore, MAO inhibition prevents serotonin breakdown and subsequently raises levels of serotonin. This feature can assist in the treatment of depression.

MB has antidepressant as well as anxiolytic activity.

Eroğlu and Cağlayan (1997) wrote *"MB acts as a direct inhibitor of NOS (nitric oxide synthase) as well as of sGC (*soluble guanylyl cyclase). *It also inactivates NO (nitric oxide) extracellularly through generation of superoxide anions. Thus, it can be speculated that NOS-NO-cGMP pathway may be involved in the antidepressant and anxiolytic actions of MB..."*

MB is of great interest to psychiatrists as it has antidepressive, anxiolytic and neuroprotective properties documented by both animal and human studies (Alda, 2019).

Deutsch et al. (1997) studied eight patients with schizophrenia who had incomplete responses to conventional medications. They completed a 4-week open-label study with a one week "on" and one week "off" protocol. The researchers noted *"A statistically significant, albeit modest, decrease in the severity of psychopathology was observed while the subjects were taking MB, and psychopathology significantly worsened when MB was discontinued."*

Naylor, Smith, and Connelly (1987) performed a study looking at MB 15 mg/day and compared with placebo in the treatment of severe depression. They concluded that MB at 15 mg/day produced a greater improvement in depression than the placebo. MB is a potent antidepressant.

Alda et al. (2017) compared 15 mgs MB (subtherapeutic "placebo") with 195 mg MB as the active treatment while maintaining lamotrigine as their primary mood stabilizer and showed that *"Methylene blue used as an adjunctive medication improved residual symptoms of depression and anxiety in patients with bipolar disorder."*

MB has multiple actions including a non-selective inhibitor of nitric oxide synthase (NOS) and guanylate cycles. Any abnormal function of the nitric oxide (NO)-cyclic guanosine monophosphate (CGMP) cascade is associated with the neurobiology of mood, depression, anxiety and psychosis. These disorders are also associated with mitochondrial dysfunction and redox imbalance, both of which MB restores.

This improves neuronal energy and inhibits the formation of superoxide. For these reasons, MB can also be useful in neurodegenerative brain diseases such as AD and Parkinson's disease.

MB is a potent MAO inhibitor which can be a reason for its antidepressant activity (Delport, Harvey, Petzer, & Petzer, 2017).

Zoellner et al. (2017) showed MB could be useful in PTSD. The researchers administered MB in association with image exposure and showed that the MB improved outcomes.

Ageing and senescence

As we have seen, MB has antioxidant properties. It is a redox agent, reducing to leucoMB then oxidising back to MB.

Mitochondrial dysfunction has been observed in many tissues, including brain, heart and skin. This is because there is increased oxidative stress.

One of the theories of ageing is the "free radical theory", where free radicals attack the tissues causing damage. Reactive oxygen species (ROS) are formed mainly in the mitochondria, though mitochondria mass decreases with ageing. Mitochondrial dysfunction leads to reduced ATP production and increased ROS production, which then further damages mitochondria. This vicious cycle causes additional damage and ageing. MB improves mitochondrial dysfunction thus breaking the damage cycle.

Mitochondrial dysfunction in the brain has been associated with neuronal loss, which has been observed in AD, Parkinson's disease, and brain injuries.

MB can cross the blood brain barrier (BBB) easily so would be ideal for the treatment of brain degeneration. MB has antioxidant properties, as well as improving mitochondrial function.

Up to this point, most of the research has been done on animal models. More research is needed, especially in humans.

Xue, Thaivalappil, and Cao (2021) reviewed the recent research and concluded that MB can be useful in neurodegeneration, memory loss, skin ageing and possibly also in the progeria – the premature ageing disease.

A major cause of skin ageing, wrinkles, pigmentation and weakened wound healing is oxidative stress. Antioxidant skin care can be an effective approach to treating ageing skin. MB is an antioxidant as well as a mitochondria support.

Xiong et al. (2017) showed a *"... potent ROS scavenging efficacy in cultured human skin fibroblasts derived from healthy donors and from patients with pro-geria ... "* They concluded that MB has a great potential for skin care.

Atamna et al. (2008) concluded that mitochondrial dysfunction and oxidative stress are the key deviations that leads to cellular senescence and ageing, and that MB can be useful in preventing this from happening.

Sarcopoenia

Sarcopoenia is a disease associated with ageing caused by a loss of skeletal muscle mass, function and strength. It interferes with the ability to perform every-day activities.
(https://aimss.org.au/research/about-musculoskel-etal-diseases/sarcopenia/ accessed 10 February 2025).

Treatment includes diet, nutrition, supplements, exercise as well as MB. As we have seen, MB acts as a mitochondrial enhancer, as an antioxidant and can improve cellular function. We can assume that if mitochondrial function is enhanced, there would be more energy, and better use of the muscles.

This makes sense! Unfortunately, there has been little research.

As seen above, MB can have a beneficial effect on ageing, which would include sarcopoenia. It would be used in addition to an exercise programme and diet, which would include more protein, and supplements.

Cancer

MB has shown some benefit in cancer treatment and prevention. The most prominent action of MB is in conjunction with photodynamic therapy.

This may sound paradoxical, but hypoxia (reduced levels of oxygen) is a characteristic feature of many tumours. Hypoxia drives proliferation, metastasis and invasion and can reduce effectiveness of many cancer treatments.

Pominova et al. (2024) utilised a mouse Lewis lung carcinoma model and used MB in a dose of 10-20 mg/kg. The researchers concluded that *"Administration of MB at 10 mg/kg shown [sic] to increase tumor oxygenation level, potentially leading to more effective antitumor therapy. However, at higher doses (20 mg/kg), MB may cause long-term decrease in oxygenation."*

This is a good example of hormesis, which is discussed later.

As we have seen, MB is a potential photodynamic substance useful in cancer therapy.

Taldaev et al. (2023) performed a systematic review on the efficacy of MB in photodynamic anticancer therapy. The researchers concluded that *"The results of the systematic review support the suggestions that photodynamic therapy with methylene blue helps against different types of cancer, including colorectal tumor, carcinoma, and melanoma. In cases of nanopharmaceutics use, a considerable increase of anticancer therapy effectiveness was observed."*

Heat shock protein 70 (HSP70) and 90 are essential for lung cancer cells to survive and to proliferate. Sanchala, Bhatt, Pethe, Shelat, and Kulkarni (2018) compared MB with novobiocin, a known HSP70 inhibitor in an *in vitro* (cell culture) and *in vivo* (mouse model) study. The researchers concluded that *"MB demonstrated potent anticancer activity in vitro and in vivo via inhibition of Hsp70..."*

Heat shock proteins (HSP) are a group of proteins that cells produce in response to stress. They were originally thought to only be produced from heat damage, hence the name. However, they were later noted to be produced from cold, UV light, and during wound healing, in fact from *any* form of stress. The cell produces HSPs to protect itself from damage. Many HSPs can promote invasiveness, metastases, block apoptosis and promote resistance to anti-cancer drugs. They also perform chaperone functions by stabilizing new proteins to ensure correct folding.

Le, Wuertz, Biel, Thompson, and Ondrey (2022) studied MB in cell cultures of oral squamous cell carcinoma (CA-9-22), oral leukoplakia (MSK-Leuk1), and immortalized keratinocytes. They used MB as a photosensitiser and showed that MB and photodynamic therapy (PTD) "... *could be a clinically significant and cost-effective treatment for oral leukoplakia and carcinoma.*"

MB has been shown to be useful in treating the complications of cancer treatment. During head-neck cancer radiation therapy, a significant side effect is a painful condition called radiation-induced oral mucositis. Roldan, Rosenthal, Koyyalagunta, Feng, and Warner (2023) showed that MB oral rinse *was "an effective and safe topical treatment for opioid-refractory oral pain from oral mucositis associated with radiation therapy for head-neck cancer."*

Grande et al. (2022) showed that MB photodynamic therapy (MB PDT) reduced a mouse model melanoma viability and induced cell death in a "... *drug and light-dose dependant manner.*"

Neurodegenerative disease

Neurodegenerative disease includes a group of diseases where the primary characteristic is neuron loss.

This group includes:

- ALS – already discussed.
- Alzheimer's disease – already discussed.
- Parkinson's disease.
- Huntington's disease.
- Multiple sclerosis (MS).
- Batten disease (Neuronal ceroid lipofuscinosis).
- Creutzfeldt–Jakob disease (Cavaliere et al., 2013).

The current treatments are largely symptomatic. The lack of specific therapies is largely due to the blood brain barrier (BBB), which keeps close to 99% of all foreign substances out of the brain (Lamptey et al., 2022).

One substance that *can* cross the BBB is MB.

As we have seen, MB has a robust effect on neuroinflammation. Also, mitochondrial dysfunction seems to be a unifying factor in the neurodegenerative diseases. So, theoretically, MB would be potentially therapeutic in all these conditions.

> Mitochondrial dysfunction seems to be a unifying factor in the neurodegenerative diseases.

Rosenkranz et al. (2021) showed that enhancing mitochondrial activity in a mouse model of MS is a promising neuroprotective strategy. This study did *not* use MB, but as we have seen, MB can cross the BBB and improve mitochondrial activity.

In a classic animal model of multiple sclerosis (MS), Wang et al. (2016) showed that MB alleviated AMPK/SIRT1 signalling which attenuated the pathological injuries to the spinal cord. MB also reduced T helper type 17 (Th 17) responses and increased regulatory T cell (Treg) responses. The researchers concluded that MB could be useful in treating autoimmune diseases and MS.

Ommati et al. (2020) showed that *"...methylene blue administration significantly improved animals' locomotor activity and mitochondrial indices in the current animal model of MS. The effects of MB on mitochondria and mitochondrial-mediated ROS formation might play a fundamental role in the protective effects of this compound."*

Atamna et al. (2008) concluded that *"Mitochondrial dysfunction and oxidative stress are thought to be key aberrations that lead to cellular senescence and aging. MB may be useful to delay mitochondrial dys-function with aging and the decrease in complex IV in Alzheimer disease."*

Smith et al. (2017) used a rat model of Parkinson's disease (PD). They showed that MB had neuroprotective properties and preserved the dopamine neurons in the substantia nigra. The researchers wrote that *"This neuroprotection did not yield a significant behavioral improvement when motor functions were measured. However, MB significantly improved attentional performance in the five-choice task designed to measure selective and sustained attention."*

Head "buckets"

"Tasmanians with Parkinson's disease have been experimenting with red and near infrared light treatment for the past few years, after being inspired by the research work of the University of Sydney's John Mitrofanis, who used red lights on mice infected with Parkinson's."

(https://www.abc.net.au/news/2019-02-24/clinical-trials-for-wearing-led-helmets-treatment-parkinsons/10836906 accessed 9 February 2025).

With the use of head "buckets" to treat Parkinson's there has been a demonstrated improvement in the disease. It may not be a cure but any improvement in the condition is worthwhile (Hamilton, El Khoury, Hamilton, Nicklason, & Mitrofanis, 2019).

This is a form of photobiomodulation (PBM).

We have already discussed photodynamic therapy (PDT), which is where a photosensitizing material (e.g. MB) is introduced and activated by light.

In contrast, photobiomodulation (PBM) is just the use of light for therapy. A simple form of PBM is helicotherapy – the use of sunlight.

Sunlight has a significant effect on health and healing.

The founder of modern nursing, Florence Nightingale (1820-1910), noted that patients not only needed fresh air but light as well, especially sunlight. She noticed that patients in rooms facing east recovered quicker than patients who were in rooms that faced in other directions or were in rooms with no windows. Sunlight has a therapeutic effect.

Before the discovery of antibiotics, doctors found that sunlight helped to treat tuberculosis (TB) with sunatoriums (sanatoriums). Patients with TB went to sanatoriums, sat in the sun, ate good food and were largely healed. This could partially be due to the production of vitamin D caused by the action of sunlight onto the skin.

Note, city people in those days were not exposed greatly to sunlight due to dingy accommodation, working long hours in factories and the current clothing restrictions. Country people were healthier and had less TB largely because they were exposed to more sunlight working outside in the fields, therefore had better vitamin D levels. They also had better, fresher food and were living in a less crowded environment.

Kearns and Tangpricha (2014) showed the importance of vitamin D in the prevention and treatment of TB.

Both MB and PBM can affect mitochondrial activity via different mechanisms, so why not combine them? Technically this is "photodynamic therapy" (PDT).

"Since MB and PBM both target mitochondria through distinct mechanisms, a therapy combining their use may be able to ameliorate the symptoms of brain disease beyond the ability of either individual therapy" (Yang, Youngblood, Wu, & Zhang, 2020).

This combination may be worthwhile to try in Parkinson's disease and may also be beneficial in Alzheimer's disease and multiple sclerosis.

See also Gonzales-Lima and Auchter, (2015).

Peripheral neuropathy

Peripheral neuropathy refers to disease or damage to the nerves outside of the CNS, i.e. the peripheral nerves (outside of the spinal cord). This may affect sensation, movement or organ dysfunction depending on which nerves are affected. Symptoms depend on whether the sensory nerves are affected, or motor nerves or autonomic nerves. Sensory symptoms include numbness, pins and needles, or excessive pain from light touch (allodynia). When motor nerves are affected, symptoms include fasciculation (muscle twitching), cramps, and muscle weakness that can affect balance and coordination. Generally, there also may be changes to skin, hair and nails. Autonomic neuropathy produces varied symptoms including bladder and bowel control, abnormal control of blood pressure and heart rate, and reduced ability to sweat.

Causes of peripheral neuropathy include diseases such as diabetes, toxins, heavy metals (lead and mercury), chemicals, which includes some antibiotics and chemotherapeutic agents (chemotherapy induced peripheral neuropathy CIPN), infections e.g. shingles, alcohol, nutritional deficiency e.g. B vitamins, and trauma.

From a theoretical point of view, we have seen that MB has antioxidant properties, neuroprotective effects, anti-inflammatory effects and pain-relieving properties, as well as being a mitochondrial support. These are good reasons to suggest that MB can be protective. Unfortunately, there is limited research.

Cirrincione et al. (2020) showed that peripheral neuropathy caused by chemotherapeutic drug paclitaxel, is largely caused by ROS and mitochondrial damage. Although this study did not include MB, we have already discussed that MB *can* protect against ROS and prevent mitochondrial damage.

Ozkul, Ozkul, and Erbas (2022) showed that MB reduces cisplatin-induced (Cisplatin – a chemotherapeutic drug) neurotoxicity in a female rat model.

Zhang, Rojas, and Gonzalez-Lima (2006) showed that MB prevents neurodegeneration in the retina caused by rotenone, an alkaloid found in the roots of certain tropical plants, used primarily as a pesticide and a fish poison.

It has been shown that *"neural firing rates significantly decreased and finally converged to zero after MB administration."* This can reduce the pain of peripheral neuropathy (Lee, Moon, Park, Suh, & Han, 2021).

As we have seen previously, MB can reduce neuroinflammation in ifosfamide CNS damage, so we can extrapolate that MB could be used in chemotherapy induced peripheral neuropathy (CIPN).

From a theoretical point of view, MB should help treat and/or prevent peripheral neuropathy from whatever cause because of its anti-inflammatory properties, its neuroprotective properties, its ability to protect against ROS damage and its mitochondrial enhancing properties.

More research is needed. On the other hand, since MB is quite safe, there is no reason NOT to use it.

However, it is important to note that high doses of MB can cause a neuropathy. Uhelski et al. (2022) showed nerve damage in a cultured rodent dorsal root ganglia *in vitro* study. Increasing MB dosages showed increasing damage. The researchers concluded that *"It is likely that MB is neuroprotective at lower doses and toxic at higher doses."*

This is related to the hormetic effect of MB. See discussion on hormesis later.

Metabolic syndrome

Metabolic syndrome (MetS) is a syndrome comprising type 2 diabetes (T2D), hypertension, dyslipidaemia and obesity. Other related conditions are Alzheimer's disease, fatty liver, polycystic ovarian syndrome (PCOS), cancer, gall stones, and a number of minor conditions, such as skin tags, acne and male vertex balding. The underlying metabolic abnormality is elevated insulin levels (hyperinsulinaemia) with an associated insulin resistance. (See my previous book **Death by Civilization**).

Approximately 20-30% of the world's population have this condition, making it one of the most common diseases today, and this probably will get worse (Saklayen, 2018).

The molecular basis of MetS is not well-known. Recent research has looked at the role of mitochondria in the pathogenesis of MetS. Mitochondrial dysfunction contributes to the oxidative stress and inflammation found in MetS (Prasun, 2020).

Mitochondrial dysfunction contributes to the oxidative stress and inflammation found in MetS.

Kwak, Park, Lee, and Lee (2010) discuss the evidence that mitochondrial dysfunction is closely linked to diabetes, including pancreatic β-cell function, insulin resistance, obesity and diabetic vascular complications. They argue that *"... mitochondrial dysfunction could be the central defect causing the abnormal glucose metabolism in the diabetic state."*

Wang and Wei (2017) showed that mitochondrial dysfunction are involved in the pathogenesis of insulin resistance and type 2 diabetes.

There is a group of proteins called sirtuins involved in metabolic regulation. Sirtuin 1 (SIRT1) activation mimics calorie restriction and nutrient utilisation. MB was studied in relation to sirtuin expression in liver function. Mice were fed on a high fat diet and MB prevented fatty liver development. MB activated SIRT1, which promoted mitochondrial biogenesis and oxygen consumption. MB may be useful in treating the fatty liver (Shin, Kim, Wu, Choi, & Kim, 2014).

There is a strong correlation between MetS and endothelial dysfunction. Endothelial dysfunction can be regarded as an early stage in the atherosclerotic process and the key that begins the process is insulin resistance (IR), with the associated inflammation. IR can cause inflammation, but inflammation can cause the IR. They are associated, they can cause each other, and both can cause endothelial dysfunction. In a diabetic rat aorta model, there were significant arterial changes which were reversed with MB. Therefore, MB can possibly be a useful treatment of endothelial dysfunction in MetS (Privistirescu et al., 2018).

Diabetic cardiomyopathy is linked to compromised mitochondrial function and ROS generation that will ultimately lead to heart failure. In a diabetic rat model, as well as in non-diabetic rat hearts, Duicu et al. (2018) showed that MB improved mitochondrial function.

There is an underlying inflammation in MetS. In the two-way process MetS causes inflammation, and inflammation is a part of insulin resistance.

Inflammation is critical to the pathogenesis and progression of MetS (Reddy, Lent-Schochet, Ramakrishnan, McLaughlin, & Jialal, 2019).

Can the cycle be broken? Can anti-inflammatory agents be used to improve insulin resistance? There is evidence that anti-inflammatories can indeed improve diabetes (Esser, Paquot, & Scheen, 2015).

"Over a hundred years ago, high doses of salicylates were shown to lower glucose levels in diabetic patients" (Shoelson, Lee, & Goldfine, 2006).

The anti-inflammatory herb, curcumin, improves PPARγ which regulates insulin sensitivity (Balakumar et al., 2023).

Another anti-inflammatory herb, cannabidiol, potentially can improve metabolic syndrome (Wiciński et al., 2023).

As we have seen, MB does have anti-inflammatory properties, so therefore, MB can be a part of the treatment of MetS. It should, however, be a part of the wholistic approach – using diet, exercise, nutrients, herbs, lifestyle, sleep, more sunshine, less stress and so on.

Cardiovascular/cerebrovascular disease

MB has been shown to have a positive effect on the vascular system, which in turn can influence heart and brain function. MB can have this action in a few ways.

As we have seen earlier, MB can improve endothelial dysfunction. MB is known to inhibit nitric oxide synthase (NOS) and guanylate cyclase, both of which are involved in the production of NO. NO has a significant role in vasodilation. Therefore, by inhibiting NOS, MB can produce a vasoconstriction which can influence blood pressure (BP) and circulation.

When there is heart failure or shock, and there is low BP, MB can increase the BP by the vasoconstriction. We have already discussed vasoplegic shock.

The effect of MB on mitochondria has already been discussed. Stimulating the mitochondria in heart failure can improve cardiac function. Berthiaume et al. (2017) showed that MB can improve cardiac function in diabetic cardiomyopathy.

With cardiac surgery, MB administered early, in the operating room rather than in recovery, improves survival and reduces the risk of major adverse events, such as vasoplegic shock.

Oktay et al. (1993) showed that MB caused a dose-dependent rise in BP in rats.

What about humans?

MB has been used to raise BP is shock situations, vasoplegic shock, septic shock, and refractory hypotension (Weissgerber, 2008). But does MB raise BP in normal people or in people who have hypertension and on medications?

In one study, Birch and Boyce (1976) reported on a rise in BP and a reduction of renal artery flow in 12 patients undergoing nephrolithotomy, after MB intravenous injection. The elevated BP only lasted for, on average, 177 seconds before returning to normal.

Note: this was in an intraoperative situation with MB given intravenously.

There is anecdotal evidence that MB can reduce BP due to the improvement in endothelial dysfunction, but it can elevate BP in others due to the NOS inhibition. Because MB can raise BP, any hypertensive patient should be monitored with regular BP checks.

Case study 2

A 68-year-old lady with mild hypertension and on medication started MB for general health purposes. She found that her BP increased, albeit to a high normal level, but she felt unwell. She felt the best with a low normal BP. This was while taking only 5 mgs (10 drops) of MB. She reduced the dose, and the BP still became elevated. She decided to stop the MB.

Chronic reduced cerebral blood flow is a risk factor for cognitive dysfunction and Alzheimer's disease. By improving mitochondrial function, MB can improve brain function.

In a rat experiment, a group of rats had both carotid arteries occluded and were compared to a group of rats who had sham surgery. The researchers concluded that *"The results suggest that MB may be beneficial for conditions involving chronic cerebral hypoperfusion, such as mild cognitive impairment, vascular dementia and Alzheimer's disease"* (Auchter, Williams, Barksdale, Monfils, & Gonzalez-Lima, 2014).

Lin et al. (2012) posited that by improving mitochondrial function with MB, it becomes an effective neuroprotectant in neurological disorders, such as Parkinson's disease and Alzheimer's disease. They concluded that *"Our results suggest that MB can enhance brain metabolism and hemodynamics ..."*

Case study 3

This is more of a combined study. Many patients have commented that since starting MB, their thinking is much clearer. They didn't specifically complain about "brain-fog" before taking MB, but after starting it, their thinking and memory became much better.

Therefore, MB can possibly be a useful remedy for anyone who has "brain-fog" for whatever reason.

Lu, Tucker, Dong, Zhao, and Zhang (2016) concluded that *"In summary, our study suggests that MB may be a promising therapeutic agent targeting neuronal cell death and cognitive deficits following transient global cerebral ischemia."*

Talley Watts et al. (2014) showed MB to be neuroprotective against mild traumatic brain injury. This may be useful in post-concussion syndrome.

Autism and ADHD

"Autism is a complex developmental disorder with an unknown etiology and without any curative treatment" (Ghanizadeh, Berk, Farrashbandi, Alavi Shoushtari, & Villagonzalo, 2013).

The above researchers reviewed all the papers about the mitochondrial electron transport chain (ETC) in autism. All the studies that were included in the studies' criteria, showed dysfunction of the ETC in autism, as well as the production of reactive oxygen species (ROS). The researchers theorised that improving the ETC in the mitochondria and reducing the ROS may improve autism.

Frye (2020) stated that *"Further research examining biomarkers of mitochondrial dysfunction and electron transport chain activity suggest that abnormalities of mitochondrial function could affect a much higher number of children with ASD [autism spectrum disorder], perhaps up to 80%."*

Valenti, de Bari, De Filippis, Henrion-Caude, and Vacca (2014) describe clinical manifestations of mitochondrial disease and how they are often present in genetic syndromes associated with intellectual disability and adaptive behaviours. The researchers discuss how dysfunctional mitochondria and ROS are involved in the pathogenesis of neurodevelopmental syndromes such as Down's syndrome, Rett syndrome, fragile X syndrome, and autism spectrum disorders.

Improving mitochondrial function and reducing ROS may improve the condition. They further write that interventions such as MB and N acetyl cysteine (NAC) are alternative electron shuttling molecules and could possibly be used as treatment.

The use of MB is suggested, as it can:

- Enter the BBB.
- Improve mitochondrial function.
- Reduce neuroinflammation.
- Reduce ROS.

Much of this is theoretical as research is very much in the early stages.

On the other hand, MB is extremely safe, and, in my opinion, it is a shame not to try it. Why wait for years before a study is done which may never be done?

Chronic fatigue syndrome (CFS)

Chronic fatigue syndrome (CFS), also known as myalgic encephalomyelitis (ME), is a long-term illness that not only causes extreme tiredness and fatigue, but other symptoms as well.

These include:

- **Fatigue**: Severe tiredness that doesn't improve with rest.
- **Sleep issues**: Unrefreshing sleep, sleep apnoea, restless legs, and nighttime muscle spasms.
- **Cognitive impairment**: Difficulty thinking, concentrating, or remembering things.

- **Pain**: Headaches, sore throats, muscle and joint pain, and tender lymph nodes.
- **Sensitivity**: Increased sensitivity to light, sound, smells, food, and medicines.
- **Gastrointestinal issues**: Irritable bowel, bloating, gas, constipation, and diarrhea.
- **Mood swings**: Anxiety and irritability.
- **Other symptoms**: Dizziness, weakness, fainting, vision problems, chills, and night sweats.

Myhill, Booth, and McLaren-Howard (2009) showed a close correlation between CFS and mitochondrial dysfunction. People with CFS describe fatigue as a lack of energy, physical and/or mental, as well as reduced endurance and poor recovery after activity.

Filler et al. (2014) posit that fatigue is a product of mitochondrial dysfunction. MB is known to support the mitochondria; therefore, MB may be a logical treatment for CFS based on the mechanism of action on the mitochondria.

Case study 4

A 40-year-old lady with chronic fatigue syndrome commented on the increase in energy and her ability to lead a more normal life since starting MB.

Fibromyalgia

In conjunction with CFS, there is another condition, fibromyalgia. There is an overlap with CFS, in some cases lots of fatigue and little pain and in other cases little fatigue and lots of pain.

People can be anywhere along that spectrum.

Fibromyalgia is described as *"... a complex multisystem physical illness, with chronic widespread pain experienced in the muscles, ligaments and/or tendons, that lasts for at least 3 months. Widespread Pain [sic] means pain in at least 3 or 4 areas of the body i.e. above and below the waist, and on both sides of the body."* (https://fibromyalgiaaustralia.org.au/patients/what-is-fibromyalgia/ accessed 19 February 2025).

Symptoms, other than pain include sleep disturbance, fatigue, musculoskeletal stiffness, and cognitive dysfunction. MB has pain relieving and anti-inflammatory properties and provides mitochondrial support and neuroinflammation actions that can all have a positive influence in the treatment of fibromyalgia.

Unfortunately, although there are many positive anecdotes, there is limited research. The studies on pain relief, mitochondrial support and neuroinflammatory actions can be extrapolated to fibromyalgia.

COVID/long COVID

COVID-19 is a coronavirus that was first identified in China in 2019. The virus spread throughout the world and the World Health Organization (WHO) declared a pandemic in March 2020. This led to a worldwide effort to contain the virus through mandatory mask wearing, lockdowns, restriction of movement, shutting down businesses, and so on. Ultimately a "vaccine" was developed and virtually forced onto the world's population. I will not get into the controversy on whether this was a natural virus, or a lab-developed virus, whether the virus was leaked or deliberately spread, or whether the measures used were appropriate. The "vaccine" was fast tracked and possibly not researched adequately. All this I will leave for others to discuss.

SARS-CoV-2 is primarily a respiratory virus and can range from a mild 'flu-like illness to an acute respiratory distress syndrome with multi-organ failure and vasoplegic shock (Emadi, Hamidi Alamdari, Attaran, & Attaran, 2024).

Scigliano and Scigliano (2021) write that anti-cytokine drugs only work on one or a few of the dozen or so cytokines involved. Other mediators of inflammation, reactive oxygen and nitrogen species are not targeted. The one substance that can address the excess production of reactive species and cytokines is MB.

The main pathological part of the COVID virus is the spike protein. The way the spike affects the cell is through the ACE2 receptor.

MB has been shown to inhibit the protein-protein interaction (PPI) between the spike protein and the ACE2 receptor, which is the first critical step of the attachment and entry of the virus into the cell.

MB can block various COVID mutants, as well as other viruses in a similar fashion, and therefore can be considered an orally bioactive small molecule antiviral (Chuang et al., 2022).

Emadi, Hamidi Alamdari, Attaran, and Attaran (2024) concluded that *"Based on studies, MB can simultaneously affect most of the host's harmful responses caused by SARS-CoV-2 infection due to its multiple properties, including anti-hypoxemia, anti-oxidant [sic], immune system modulator, and antiviral. The use of MB is associated with a reduction in the possibility of getting infection, and mortality, and can be used as a safe, effective, cheap, and available treatment option with minimal side effects for the clinical management of COVID-19."*

After the COVID pandemic, a new disease developed, the so called "long COVID". This is characterised by persistent symptoms, in a timeframe of months, after the resolution of an acute COVID infection.

The estimate is that about three percent of people in the UK have "long COVID", and in approximately fifty percent of "long COVID" sufferers, the symptoms fit the criteria for myalgic encephalomyelitis (ME), also known as chronic fatigue syndrome (CFS). Symptoms include:

General symptoms

- Tiredness or fatigue that interferes with daily life.
- Symptoms that get worse after physical or mental effort.
- Fever.

Respiratory and heart symptoms

- Difficulty breathing or shortness of breath.
- Coughing.
- Chest pain.
- Fast-beating or pounding heart (also known as heart palpitations).

Neurological symptoms

- Difficulty thinking or concentrating (sometimes referred to as "brain fog").
- Headaches.
- Sleep problems.
- Dizziness when you stand up (light-headedness).
- Pins-and-needles.
- Change in smell or taste.

- Depression or anxiety.

Digestive symptoms

- Diarrhea.
- Stomach pain.
- Constipation.

Other symptoms

- Joint or muscle pain.
- Rash.
- Changes in menstrual cycle.

(https://www.cdc.gov/covid/long-term-effects/long-covid-signs-symptoms.html accessed 5 Feb 2025).

"Emerging evidence has pointed to mitochondrial dysfunction as a potential underpinning mechanism contributing to the persistence and diversity of long COVID symptoms" (Molnar et al., 2024).

As many of the symptoms of "long COVID" seem to relate to mitochondrial dysfunction, it would therefore be logical to consider MB as an appropriate choice of treatment, considering the safety profile of MB.

MISCELLANEOUS CONDITIONS

Burning mouth syndrome

Burning mouth syndrome is a disabling condition where there is spontaneous pain felt in the mouth and gums without any obvious mucosal abnormality. Lecor et al. (2020) used a 0.5% MB mouth rinse, for 5 minutes, three times a day for seven days. After seven days the pain was significantly reduced by two thirds and almost absent at 3- and 6-month review.

POTS syndrome

Postural orthostatic tachycardia syndrome (POTS) is a condition that causes an abnormally fast heart rate when standing or sitting up.

It's a type of dysautonomia, which is a disorder of the autonomic nervous system.

Dysautonomia is a failure of the autonomic nervous system to regulate certain body functions, such as heart rate, blood pressure, temperature, respiration, digestion, etc. One example of this is POTS.

POTS has been known for some time, and can be triggered by viral or bacterial infections, including SARS Cov-19. POTS has been associated with "long COVID".

There is evidence that dysautonomia is related to mitochondrial dysfunction.

"Disturbances in autonomic nervous system function have been reported to occur in patients suffering from mitochondrial cytopathies" (Kanjwal, Karabin, Kanjwal, Saeed, & Grubb, 2010).

Note – mitochondrial cytopathy refers to failure of mitochondrial function – i.e. mitochondrial dysfunction.

Many functional diseases, including POTS and interstitial cystitis, can also be related to mitochondrial dysfunction, and many, if investigated by looking at the genetics, can be related to a genetic abnormality.

(http://longislandeds.com/slides/diConfprivate/Boles.DysautomiaAndMitoCME.pdf accessed 16 March 2025).

There is some evidence that MB can help dysautonomia, and therefore POTS.

Unfortunately, there are no specific studies looking at MB and POTS.

There is only anecdotal evidence.

Dr Scott Sherr is an American Board-Certified internal medicine physician who has, in a podcast on a POTS advocacy website, described his work with MB and POTS. He has also done many podcasts on this topic and can easily be found by searching the internet.

(https://www.standinguptopots.org/potscast/e235-xxx accessed 16 March 2025).

MB is very safe. And since there may be associated fatigue, brain fog, etc. for which MB can be helpful it could be used as part of the treatment for this condition – not necessarily the only treatment.

Priapism

Priapism is named after Priapus, the Greek God of fertility, gardening, and lust. The Romans later incorporated this deity into their culture, and artistic representations often show him with a huge erect penis.

"Priapism is defined as a full or partial erection lasting longer than 4 hours after sexual stimulation and orgasm or is unrelated to sexual stimulation" (Yücel, Salabaş, Ermeç, & Kadıoğlu, 2017).

Intracavernous injection for the treatment of erectile dysfunction, e.g. a mixture of papaverine, phentolamine and prostaglandin E1, (colloquially referred to as the "prick in the dick"!) can have a side effect of priapism.

"The authors recommend intravenous methylene blue for the treatment of priapism" (Hübler, Szántó, & Könyves, 2003).

"These results confirm that MB is a safe and highly effective treatment agent for short-term pharmacologically induced priapism. The application of MB shows virtually no significant side effects compared to the systemic and local complications induced by alpha-adrenergic agonists" (Martínez Portillo, Hoang-Boehm, Weiss, Alken, & Jünemann, 2001).

Of course, MB treatment of priapism should be done in a hospital, as the treatment involves intravenous MB.

Post concussion syndrome

Post concussion syndrome (PCS) is a syndrome of varied symptoms. As the name suggests, it occurs after a concussion, i.e. trauma to the head. The trauma can be very mild to severe and can be referred to as traumatic brain injury (TBI). For the majority, the symptoms of concussion resolve over days to a week; however, in a minority the symptoms can persist for months to years.

"The clinical consequences of concussion may be best conceptualized as two multidimensional disorders: (1) a constellation of acute symptoms termed early-phase posttraumatic disorder (commonly headache, dizziness, imbalance, fatigue, sleep disruption, impaired cognition, photo- and phonophobia); and (2) late-phase posttraumatic disorder, consisting of somatic, emotional, and cognitive symptoms" (Dwyer & Katz, 2018).

Psychosocial factors may have an influence on the chronic phase.

"Risk factors for development of a late-phase disorder include a high early symptom burden (e.g., headache, fatigue), a history of multiple concussions, psychiatric conditions (anxiety, depression), longer duration of unconsciousness or amnesia, and younger age" (Dwyer & Katz, 2018).

In a rat brain trauma model, Genrikhs et al. (2020), showed that a MB injection, thirty minutes after injury, reduced the impairment of the motor functions of the limbs. They also showed that monthly MB given for six months, was the most effective. MB is known to have antioxidant properties and does cross the blood brain barrier (BBB).

In another rat brain trauma model, Talley Watts et al. (2014) concluded *"... MB treatment minimized lesion volume, behavioral deficits, and neuronal degeneration following mild TBI."*

Isaev, Genrikhs, and Stelmashook (2024) commented that the neurodegenerative processes can continue after the acute phase of TBI and ischaemia, with development of brain atrophy with dementia. This is like the neurodegeneration characteristic of Alzheimer's disease (AD). The researchers further state that there are many processes involved, including oxidative stress, inflammation, glial activation, BBB dysfunction, and excessive autophagy. MB can address these processes. The researchers continue *"This drug [i.e. MB] can have an antiapoptotic and anti-inflammatory effect, activate autophagy, inhibit the aggregation of proteins with an irregular shape, inhibit NO synthase, and bypass impaired electron transfer in the respiratory chain of mitochondria."*

They conclude that *"In recent years, this drug [i.e. MB] has attracted great interest as a potential treatment for a number of neurodegenerative disorders, including the effects of TBI, ischemia, and AD."*

Although many of these studies are done on a rat brain trauma model and do not specifically mention post-concussion syndrome (PCS), they do exemplify that MB can help the brain recover after head trauma. Again, do not forget that MB can treat some of the other symptoms of PCS.

Pain relief

As we have seen, MB has local anaesthetic properties. MB injection during knee replacement, after perianal surgery and after costal cartilage harvesting produces pain relief.

Lee and Han (2021) showed that MB reduces pain in three ways.

1. MB downregulates NO (this we have seen) but under pathological conditions, NO is overexpressed and contributes to inflammation as a pro-inflammatory mediator. Suppressing NO reduces inflammation.
2. MB reduces voltage-gated sodium channels (VGSCs). It, therefore, reduces the firing rates of afferent nerve fibres, thus impeding pain transmission.
3. MB hinders or damages nerve connection to tissues; this is referred to as denervation. This in effect makes nerve fibres incapable of sensing pain.

MB can be used in the treatment of discogenic low back pain. MB is injected into the degenerate lumbar disc. This technique has shown long term pain relief. There have been a meta-analysis and random placebo-controlled trials. Most have shown positive benefits (Gupta, Radhakrishna, Chankowsky, & Asenjo, 2012; Deng et al., 2021; Waardenburg, de Meij, Brouwer, Van Zundert, & van Kuijk, 2022; Peng, Pang, Wu, Zhao, & Song, 2010; Guo, Ding, Liu, & Yang, 2019).

However, Kallewaard et al. (2019) did not show benefit.

MB can help relieve the pain of a full-thickness rectal prolapse, which can be a very painful condition.

Miralles, López-Bas, Díaz-Alejo, and Roldan (2024) report on a case of an elderly patient with pain associated with chronic rectal prolapse. Surgery was ruled out, and systemic analgesics gave no relief. Topical MB 0.1% solution was applied to the prolapsed rectum, and the patient experienced immediate and long-lasting pain relief. The MB was applied 12 hourly, as needed.

In a mouse model, Dondas et al. (2013) administered painful stimuli to two groups of mice: one group given MB and the other a saline placebo. The researchers concluded that *"chronic administration of MB has analgesic effects on acute nociception as well as on the orofacial inflammatory pain."*

In a rat model, Lee, Moon, Park, Suh and Han (2021) showed that MB significantly decreased neural firing rates after MB administration in rats. They con-cluded that *"Therefore, these results demonstrate that MB lessens pain by significantly weakening neural ex-citability, which implies a strong possibility that this dye may be developed as a pain-relieving medication in the future."*

As we have seen, MB has anti-inflammatory prop-erties as well as pain relieving properties. So, in practice, MB can be a part of treatment for any chronic pain con-ditions, including fibromyalgia, chronic pain syndromes and possibly even endometriosis.

Infected wounds

Shen et al. (2020) treated infected wounds with MB and photodynamic therapy (MB-PDT). *"After an average of 4 PDT session, infected wounds of all the pa-tients healed. The treatment also showed an excellent cosmetic effect."* The researchers concluded that *"MB-PDT has a great healing effect on infected wounds, and it is a safe, cheap and active clinical therapy."*

Chronic wounds

Cesar et al. (2022) report on a series of cases of a poorly healing chronic ulcer. A 1% MB solution was ap-plied to the ulcer and irradiated with a red LED diode light source weekly. The wound showed significant secretion reduction, no local reaction and no adverse reactions. *"The results were satisfactory, with significant wound size reduction, and a decrease in aspects indicative of infection including odor, presence of exudates, and purulence."*

This technique can be used for diabetic foot ulcers, venous leg ulcers and pressure ulcers.

Chronic anal fissures

Chronic anal fissures (CAFs) are the second most common anorectal disease. Symptoms include pain and bleeding. Acute fissures generally heal within six weeks, but if not healed by then they can become chronic, and these are often difficult to treat. Lobascio et al. (2025) used MB with a glyceryl trinitrate-based cream to treat chronic anal fissures in a randomised phase 2 trial. They concluded that *"Methylene blue-based ointments could be a new and innovative treatment for the non-operative management and healing of CAFs."*

Skin diseases

Salah, Samy, and Fadel (2009) used a MB hydrogel in conjunction with photodynamic therapy (PTD) on resistant psoriatic plaques. The researchers concluded that *"The results are encouraging to accept MB as a photosensitizer for PDT and as a safe and effective method for treatment of selected cases of resistant localized psoriasis."*

Fadel, Salah, Samy, and Mona (2009) used liposomal MB hydrogel in conjunction with PDT to treat mild to moderate acne vulgaris.

Aghahosseini, Arbabi-Kalati, Fashtami, Fateh, and Djavid (2006) used MB with PTD (MB-PDT) to treat oral lichen planus (OLP). They concluded that *"MB-PDT blue seems to be an effective alternative treatment for control of OLP."*

Sadaksharam, Nayaki, and Selvam (2012) came to a similar conclusion.

Waingade, Medikeri, and Rathod (2022) compared MB-PTD with corticosteroid therapy in treating OLP. They concluded that both were effective. They continued by saying that MB-PTD is an alternative option when steroids are contraindicated.

Lichen sclerosis is a chronic inflammatory skin condition of unknown cause; though there is a thought it may be autoimmune.

The condition mostly affects the anal area, and the genitals, vulva or penis. Without treatment, scarring will develop which would interfere with sexual intercourse, urination, and defecation. A long-term consequence is the increased chance of developing skin cancer.

Belotto et al. (2017) compared 1) standard treatment with steroids, 2) MB-PDT, and 3) with just red-light therapy; photobiomodulation (PBM). The MB was not applied to the lichen sclerosis lesions but injected into eight points around the vulval area.

The steroid group showed 60% remission, but the complications of skin atrophy, scarring and hypopigmentation were irreversible. The MB-PDT group had good response, whilst the PBM alone had negligible effect.

Chang and Weinstein (1975) used MB and light exposure to treat eczema herpeticum.

Alberdi and Gómez (2020) used MB-PTD to treat pityriasis versicolour (PV). PV is a fungal infection caused by a yeast from the Malassezia genus. This results in discoloured patches on the skin, which may be lighter or darker than the surrounding skin.

The researchers applied a 2% MB solution to the lesions for three minutes, then a red LED lamp was placed 100 mm from the skin for 10 minutes. They concluded that *"Six sessions of MB/PDT spaced at 14-day intervals are sufficient for the treatment for PV in healthy patients."*

In a systematic review, Shen, Jemec, Arendrup, and Saunte (2020) showed that MB-PTD was efficacious with complete cure rates of 70-80% of superficial fungal infections.

MB-PDT can treat onychomycosis – Trichophyton rubrum fungal infection of the nails. MB is painted onto the nails and irradiated with a red LED light (Souza, Souza, & Botelho 2014; Alberdi & Gómez, 2019).

Case study 5

An elderly gentleman with multiple medical conditions and on an extensive list of medications presented with severe onychomycosis of all his toes. All his toenails were grossly thickened and uncomfortable. As he was on multiple medications, I was reluctant to add another, an antifungal. So, I suggested he paint his toenails with MB and expose them to the sun. The next time I saw him he had very trendy bright blue toenails! After three months the toenails were very much improved. The nails were still not normal but the thickened onycomycotic toenails were very much less, and he was much more comfortable.

In another study, MB was painted onto the nails and then illuminated with a light source. Fifty three out of 62 patients responded well without any pain or burning sensation (Tardivo, Wainwright, & Baptista, 2015).

Bowornsathitchai et al. (2021) showed MB-PDT to be superior to 5% amorolfine nail lacquer for non-dermatophyte onychomycosis, such as Fusarium spp., Aspergillus spp., and yeasts.

MB has been shown to be very helpful in intractable pruritus ani. The MB is injected intradermally into the perianal skin (Sutherland, Faragher, & Frizelle, 2009). Kim, Kim, and Lee (2019) showed a high symptom improvement rate, and a low recurrence rate; 7.5% after 3 years.

Conventional photodynamic therapy (PDT) may be inconvenient for some; not everyone can have access to the LED red light, so an alternative is "daylight photodynamic therapy" (DL PDT). This is basically the use of sunlight. The MB photosensitiser is applied to the lesion and then is exposed to sunlight. The downside of this is that sunlight dosing cannot be standardised, and sunlight may not always be present.

In a randomised double-blind placebo-controlled study, Fathy, Asaad, and Rasheed (2017) used DL PDT with 10% MB gel and compared with placebo to treat plane warts. One hundred percent showed no response in the placebo group, while in the active group 65% showed complete clearance, 10% showed good response and 25% showed poor response.

Beshay, El Kahky, and Mohammad (2023) treated molluscum contagiosum (MC) with DL PDT and MB. They concluded that the DL PDT with MB is effective in clearing MC.

MC is a viral skin infection producing pinkish lesions with a characteristic dimple in the middle.

Chang, Fiumara, and Weinstein (1975) treated genital herpes with topical MB and light exposure. The lesions were eradicated in seventy percent of cases. However, the authors state the recurrence was not prevented or reduced, although the lesions healed quicker.

Tardivo et al. (2005) concluded that MB PDT has been shown to treat basal cell carcinoma, Kaposi's sarcoma, melanoma, virus and fungal infections.

Tardivo, Del Giglio, Paschoal, and Baptista (2006) report a case study of a patient with multiple Kaposi's sarcoma lesions that were treated unsuccessfully with chemotherapy. The researchers then used MB PDT. MB was injected into the lesions and light applied. There was complete remission with excellent cosmetic results.

In a mouse model of squamous cell carcinoma using MB PDT, Silva et al. (2018) showed that *"In the squamous cell carcinoma group, photodynamic therapy reduced tumor size and cell proliferation and raised cytokine levels. In normal skin, it decreased cell prolif-eration and collagen quantity and increased apoptosis and blood vessel numbers."*

From a theoretical point of view, MB plus or minus PDT can be used for shingles and post-herpetic neural-gia, due to its anti-viral, anti-inflammatory, and analge-sic properties. If it can be used on herpes labialis and herpes genitalis, why not shingles?

Cui, Zhang, Zhang, and Ma (2016) treated severe acute thoracic shingles with intracutaneous MB injec-tion. The researchers concluded that *"Intradermal injec-tion of methylene blue can effectively shorten the disease course, reduce the pain intensity and prevent the devel-opment of postherpetic neuralgia in elderly patients with herpes zoster."*

What about topical MB?

What if we add dimethyl sulfoxide (DMSO) to the MB? DMSO is a carrier molecule which would increase the absorption of the MB into the tissues. DMSO also has anti-inflammatory and analgesic properties.

Is it worth trying? Why not?

MB and DMSO are quite safe!

There are many conventional treatments for shin-gles and post-herpetic neuralgia. The anti-viral medication only works if used in the first 72 hours of the symptoms. What if you miss this timeframe?

Some people may not want conventional treatment. Their philosophy is one of having a more natural treatment. One non-conventional treatment for shingles that works is intravenous vitamin C (Liu, Wang, Xiong, Zhang, & Fang, 2020; Schencking et al., 2012).

One issue with MB is that, depending on concentration, it can stain the skin for a time. A 1% solution can last for hours to days. A dilution of 0.1% may still be effective and will stain less. Obviously, a blue stain on the face may cause issues, while stains on other parts of the body can be hidden by clothing.

The MB can be applied directly to the lesion, whether it is a wart, herpes lesion, molluscum contagiosum, and so on, and the light applied, whether red LED light or laser, or daylight.

However, there can possibly be embarrassing issues when exposing genital lesions to the sunlight!

What if leucoMB is used?

It has no colour and does not stain – unfortunately, leucoMB does not have the same photosensitising properties as MB; *"... the formed colorless leucomethylene blue has negligible photodynamic activity"* (Seong & Kim, 2015).

Radiation-induced oral mucositis

Radiotherapy for cancer to the neck and head can produce a painful oral mucositis that generally fails conventional treatment. MB oral rinse has been shown to be a safe and effective treatment for this painful condition (Roldan, Rosenthal, Koyyalagunta, Feng, & Warner, 2023).

Lyme disease

Lyme disease is an infectious disease caused by *Borrelia burgdorferi* and related species. A common co-infection is with *Bartonella* species. The transmission is via a tick bite.

Symptoms are:

Early localised stage (days to weeks after bite)

- Rash, especially the "target lesion" or "bull's eye lesion" that appears in 70-80% of cases.
- Influenza-like symptoms.
- Early disseminated stage (weeks to months after bite)
- Multiple rashes.

Neurological symptoms

- Bell's palsy.

- Nerve pain; tingling numbness.
- Meningitis-like symptoms; neck stiffness, headache.

Heart symptoms

- Palpitations.
- AV block leading to irregular heartbeat.

Late disseminated stage (months to years after bite)

- Chronic arthritis.

Neurological issues

- Brain fog.
- Memory issues.
- Poor concentration.
- Severe fatigue.

Post-treatment Lyme disease syndrome/chronic Lyme

These symptoms can persist despite antibiotic treatment.

- Immune system dysfunction.
- Inflammation.

Lyme disease occurs mainly in the USA, Europe and Asia. According to the Australian government and Australian health authorities, Lyme disease does *not* exist in Australia, as there have not been any confirmed finding of *Borrelia burgdorferi* in Australian ticks.

However, there are Australians who report Lyme-like symptoms after a tick bite. The controversy is that this may represent a similar illness caused by a different *Borrelia* species. However, not everyone bitten by a tick gets this disease. Why? Researchers are trying to find a cause but till now, none has been found.

Nevertheless, Australians do suffer from a similar illness. In 2018, the Australian Department of Health renamed this disease. It was no longer called Lyme-like disease but now called it debilitating symptom complexes attributed to ticks (DSCATT).

Why do I discuss Lyme disease?

This is because MB can be part of the treatment; it may be experimental and not accepted by mainstream medicine, but functional medicine doctors have been using MB to treat their patients.

MB has been shown to have,

- Antimicrobial effects, specifically against *Borrelia* and *Bartonella* (Feng et al., 2015; Li et al., 2019).
- Biofilm disruption (Zheng, Ma, Li, Shi, & Zhang, 2020). One idea is that the bacteria enter a stationary phase or form a biofilm which make it more difficult to eradicate.
- Mitochondrial support.
- Neuroprotective properties.

- Anti-inflammatory properties.

Although not the whole treatment, MB can be part of Lyme disease, and Lyme-like disease treatment protocols.

Mast cell activation syndrome (MCAS)

Mast cells are the cells responsible for immediate allergy reactions. The cells make and store chemicals, such as histamine and prostaglandins, known as mediators, in granules inside the cell. When an IgE allergen antibody interacts with receptors on the cell surface, a reaction occurs, and these chemicals are released causing an immediate allergic reaction. Some of these chemicals are fast acting and some are slow. Mast cells can also be activated by some medications, infections, and insect or reptile venoms. These are normal reactions.

For yet unknown reasons, mast cells can become defective and release the chemicals because of abnormal internal signals.

"However, there are also abnormal conditions, in which this process is not regulated and, like mast cell activation syndrome (MCAS), causes manifestations in different organ systems in the body. Therefore, MCAS is a disorder that should be considered and diagnosed clinically with specific signs and symptoms of activation in

111

individuals with skin, gastrointestinal, cardiovascular, respiratory, and neurological system involvement" (Özdemir, Kasımoğlu, Bak, Sütlüoğlu, & Savaşan, 2024).

Symptoms include unexplained episodes of severe swelling, urticaria (hives), diarrhoea, vomiting, low blood pressure, shortness of breath, cognitive dysfunction, chronic pain, flushing and itching. Another issue is that the person may start to develop reactions to foods, medication, herbs, and nutrients. This can become very frustrating, for both doctor and patient as they react to everything that is tried. The symptoms are like those of an allergic reaction, but there are no clear triggers. The reaction can be severe enough to cause anaphylaxis, which can be life threatening. Although this condition is like an allergic reaction, it is not. For unknown reasons, the mast cells degranulate releasing the mediating factors.

Some causes include environmental toxins such as mould and mercury; thus, the condition is becoming more common in our toxic, polluted world.

MCAS is often found in association with other conditions such as irritable bowel syndrome (IBS), "long COVID", Ehlers-Danlos syndrome (EDS), fibromyalgia, chronic fatigue syndrome (CFS), and postural orthostatic tachycardia syndrome (POTS).

There is a related condition – called mastocytosis, where the number of mast cells is greatly increased. The most common cause is a genetic mutation of the gene that controls the growth and activity of mast cells. It is considered a rare disorder.

Although not generally established, MB can have a role in treating MCAS. There are no specific studies, but there is much anecdotal evidence.

- MB can stabilise the mast cell, inhibiting degranulation.
- MB has anti-inflammatory action and antioxidant properties which may counteract the oxidative stress generally found with MCAS.
- MB has NO modulating properties. Some with MCAS have been shown to have issues with NO regulation.
- MB has neuroprotective properties. MCAS is associated with cognitive dysfunction, therefore may help in MCAS brain fog.

MCAS is associated with sensitivity to medications, so it is important to start with a much lower dose than usual. Of course, all the other precautions should be adhered to.

While on the topic of MCAS, another very useful herb to try is cannabidiol (CBD) oil. This also has mast cell membrane stabilising properties, is anti-inflammatory, notably reduces tumour necrosis factor alpha (TNFα) – a pro-inflammatory cytokine, and interleukin 6 (Il-6) - a cytokine, which is elevated in MCAS. This influences the endocannabinoid system which regulates the immune system, may reduce histamine effects on the gut, and has anti-itch effects on the skin.

Yang et al. (2023) showed in a mouse model that cannabidiol inhibits IgE mediated mast cell degranulation and anaphylaxis.

There are conventional treatments for MCAS. MB and CBD can be a part of these.

Also note that, as previously mentioned, MB can be used for the conditions associated with MCAS – fibromyalgia, CFS, POTS, and so on.

Nasal allergy

There is a relationship between NO and allergies. Most of the NO effects are mediated by guanylate cyclase (GC). MB inhibits the activity of GC when applied to the nasal mucosa in allergic rhinitis patients.

Kawamoto, Watanabe, Yajin, and Kouro (1999) showed that not only did MB inhibit the nasal provocation of some allergens but also showed that MB potentially inhibited the release of chemical mediators, as well as having a non-specific effect on nasal hypersensitivity.

Unfortunately, there are no other studies, so we can only speculate that a MB nasal spray could be used to treat nasal allergies.

Endometriosis

Endometriosis is a condition, usually resulting in pain and dysmenorrhea, which is characterized by the abnormal occurrence of functional endometrial tissue outside the uterus. Unfortunately, it is quite common, approximately 1 in 7 women is affected by endometriosis. Fifty percent develop fertility issues and one third have mental health problems. Overall, Australia spends A$9.7 billion per year on this condition.

The condition is related to multiple factors including epigenetic, environmental, hormonal, immune, inflammatory, and gastro-intestinal issues.

Unfortunately, there are no specific studies looking at treating endometriosis with MB, however, as we have seen, MB has anti-inflammatory and anti-fibrotic activity, as well as antioxidant and pain-relieving properties. These all should, theoretically, help the condition, suggesting that MB should be a *part* of the treatment of this complex, multifactorial condition.

Endometriosis also has various cognitive symptoms, which can be primary or secondary; "brain fog", fatigue, anxiety and depression and MB could help with these.

MB has been used for many years during laparoscopic examination. It is particularly useful when used as a stain *"to detect the loss of peritoneal integrity in patients with pelvic pain and suspected endometriosis"* (Lessey, Higdon, Miller, & Price, 2012).

HOW TO TAKE METHYLENE BLUE

Hormesis

Hormesis is a term referring to the ability of a substance to have a positive effect at a low dose, while having an opposite negative effect at a high dose. Basically, there is a biphasic effect: Safe in low doses, dangerous in high doses (Mattson, 2007). MB has this property (Bruchey & Gonzales-Lima, 2008).

Small doses of MB are safe and beneficial. These small doses can be used daily, and continuously. Large doses can be possibly dangerous. Intermediate doses may be non-effective.

However, note that in life-threatening situations, e.g. methaemoglobinaemia, a higher dose of MB needs to be given intravenously. This is a one-off or perhaps a second dose may be needed. High doses for a long time can possibly have a negative effect.

Dosage

As alluded to above, dosage is important. An excessive dose can cause an opposite, therefore, unwanted, effect.

Intravenous dosage

For life-death situations, high doses of MB are needed and are generally given intravenously, though only as a once or twice off dose. For example, in methaemoglobinaemia, the recommended dose is based on body weight – 1-2 mg/kg/dose, up to a maximum of 7 mg/kg/dose. This is to be administered intravenously over a 5-minute period. A repeat dose can be given, if needed, after one hour.

Similar doses are required for vasoplegic shock not responding to other measures.

Paradoxically, MB in doses greater than 7mg/kg, given quickly over 2-3 hours can *cause* methaemoglobinaemia. This is a good example of hormesis.

(https://www.poisonsinfo.health.qld.gov.au/for-health-professionals/antidote-stocking-recommendations/methylene-blue accessed 8 February 2025).

Intradermal/intra-articular injection

MB has been shown to act effectively as a local anaesthetic. A 1% sterile MB solution can be injected intradermally to treat chronic pain e.g. post herpetic neuralgia, and to relieve pain post operatively, e.g. post haemorrhoidectomy. In a mouse model, MB was injected into joints to treat osteoarthritis. MB can be injected into intravertebral discs to treat chronic back pain.

Oral dosage

Multiple dosing protocols exist. Many authors suggest a dose of 0.5 – 3 mg/kg, however, this can be a big dose – this would mean that an 80 kg person can take up to 240 mg of MB! This dosage regime is probably related to the IV dose protocols.

For general use, I would follow the advice of Dr Joseph Mercola, who suggests an oral dose of 3-5 mgs, irrespective of weight. He believes that anything more than this is excessive and unnecessary. In this context "Less is more"!

You can find Dr Mercola's information here. (https://media.mercola.com/ImageServer/Public/2024/October/PDF/methylene-blue-benefits-side-effects-pdf.pdf accessed 8 February 2025).

Some practitioners advocate a "loading dose", giving a slightly higher dose for the first two weeks, then reducing to the maintenance dose of 5 mgs daily.

Either way, the "start low and go slow" protocol should be followed. Start low, for example 3 mgs (equivalent to 6 drops of the 1% solution) and slowly increase to 10 drops (equivalent to 5 mg of the 1% solution). This can be continued up to 15 mgs.

An internet search regarding dosage is very confusing. There is a multitude of suggestions for maximum dosage. The best protocol is "start low, go slow and keep low".

> Start low, go slow and keep low.

Everyone is different, so when treating a specific condition, we can use the signs and symptoms to determine the dose. Slowly increase the dose until there is improvement – then stay on that dose. If a 5 mg dose does not improve the situation, then the dose can be increased slowly. The bottom line is that the dosage should be more on the low side than on the high side.

When using MB for long-term prevention, e.g. Alzheimer's disease, then the 5 mgs dosage is probably adequate.

A once-a-day dose is adequate, though some sites say a twice a day dose is needed.

Generally, MB comes as a 1% solution (10 mgs/ml). Twenty drops are equivalent to 1 ml, (therefore 10 drops are equivalent to half a ml, which equals 5 mgs) to be taken daily in a glass of water.

If larger doses are required, compounding pharmacists can make MB capsules at any required dosage, but high doses are not generally necessary. Beware of the hormetic effect.

There is a recommendation to take a day off every week to prevent accumulation.

For treatment of malaria, oral doses of 10-12 mg/kg/day are used, but only for short-term use.

Once MB is added to water, it turns a beautiful blue colour. If you drink this, your tongue will turn blue! There are memes on the internet with people showing their blue tongues!

To prevent this, mix a quarter of a teaspoon of ascorbic acid powder into the water first, then add the MB. (It **must be ascorbic acid**, not sodium ascorbate, or calcium ascorbate). Within a matter of minutes, the dark blue colour will change to an almost clear liquid.

What has happened is that the MB (which is in the oxidised form) is reduced to clear leucoMB by the ascorbic acid.

You can now drink the clear liquid without getting a blue tongue. Your urine will still be blue though!

Topical dosage

MB can be administered topically as a solution, cream, or a gel. A 1% MB solution will stain the skin bright blue for an extended period. For topical use, a 0.1% solution is adequate, especially if using a light source, photodynamic therapy (PDT), but it can still stain the skin blue. An even more dilute solution is needed.

A 0.01% solution will cause minimal staining and can be applied locally to acne, warts, and even painful areas, such as neuralgia and tendonitis as a pain relief. To enhance the action, DMSO can be added to increase absorption. Red light therapy can also be used.

MB cream can also be used as a cosmetic and for anti-ageing purposes. It can be purchased on-line in Australia, though note the legal aspects that I will discuss later.

Obviously applying a bright blue dye to the face can be embarrassing, but if applied to the body, it can be hidden by clothing. A 0.01% solution has minimal colouring and can be used on the face.

Pharmacokinetics

MB is well absorbed after an oral dose, though this can be variable. Estimates show that 53% to 97% (average 74%) is absorbed. Once absorbed, there is some first-pass metabolism and peripheral conversion to leucoMB. MB is excreted in bile, faeces and urine; approximately 40% is unchanged, hence the blue urine. Peak serum level is achieved in 1-2 hours. Intravenously the peak is reached in 30 minutes. Half-life of an oral dose can be from 5 to 6.5 hours. The half-life of an intravenous dose is around 24 hours. MB is 94% protein bound.

(https://www.medicine.com/drug/methylene-blue/hcp accessed 20 February 2025).

Precautions

MB is relatively safe but there are situations where it should *not* be taken.

Who cannot take MB?

As we shall see, any person taking a selective serotonin reuptake inhibitor (SSRI), serotonin-norepinephrine reuptake inhibitors (SNRI) or monoamine oxidase inhibitor (MAOI) medication should not take MB as a serotonin syndrome may develop.

Glucose 6 phosphate dehydrogenase (G6PD) deficiency is a genetic disorder where the blood cells break down if exposed to certain triggers. Often called "favism" because one of the triggers is the fava bean (broad bean). Since it is an X linked recessive gene, the condition occurs nearly exclusively in males, though there are some double X recessive females.

Once the red blood cells (RBC) start to break down, this leads to a haemolytic anaemia. Treatment of an acute haemolytic anaemia would be a blood transfusion. The mainstay of treatment is prevention - to avoid the triggers.

One of the triggers can be MB.

In a study of children in Burkina Faso by Müller et al. (2013), children with uncomplicated malaria were treated with MB. Two children with G6PD (one a heterozygous and one homozygous) were found in the MB group, and the researchers commented that the reduction of haemoglobin was minor. They concluded that *"This effect appears to be of limited clinical relevance but needs to be monitored."*

Pregnancy and breastfeeding. There is very little data, so the best approach is to avoid.

MB had been used to inject into the amniotic sac to diagnose ruptured membranes. This intra-amniotic injection has been shown to cause problems, including haemolytic anaemia, hyperbilirubinaemia, and methaemoglobinaemia in the newborn (McEnerney & McEnerney, 1983).

Forty-six exposures have been reported during pregnancy in general, and this resulted in three malformed infants, so there may be a possible association. (https://doctorlib.org/pregnancy/drugs-pregnancy-lactation/719.html Accessed 10 August 2025).

MB is suggested to treat methaemoglobinaemia in pregnancy. However, note that *"The benefits of treatment in all patients, especially in those who are pregnant, must outweigh the inherent risks of the therapies used to treat methemoglobinemia"* (Grauman Neander, Loner, & Rotoli, 2018).

It is also wise to avoid MB in neonates and the very young.

"When in doubt, don't."
Benjamin Franklin (1706–1790)

Since MB is eliminated through the kidneys, it follows that if there is kidney disease, with a reduction of kidney function, the dosage will need to be reduced.

There is some liver metabolism of MB, therefore liver disease/ compromised liver function may determine if a smaller dose is given. Liver function would need to be monitored.

This generally would only apply to large doses, especially intravenously. The small oral doses that I recommend would probably not be an issue, however, there will need to be constant monitoring.

Serotonin syndrome

Serotonin syndrome is caused by elevated levels of serotonin in the body. This is mainly caused by medication, especially with combinations of medications that raise serotonin. MB is a monoamine oxidase inhibitor (MAOI). This enzyme metabolises serotonin. If this enzyme is inhibited, then the levels of serotonin do not reduce, but increase. Selective serotonin reuptake inhibitor (SSRIs) medications (examples escitalopram, sertraline, fluoxetine) are designed to elevate serotonin levels to treat depression. If a person is taking an SSRI and then starts to take MB, the serotonin levels can become *too* high causing the serotonin syndrome. Symptoms of serotonin syndrome include:

- Anxiety.
- Confusion.
- Dilated pupils.
- Fever.
- Flushing or paleness.
- Headache.
- High blood pressure.
- Irregular heartbeat.
- Muscle rigidity.
- Poor coordination.
- Profuse sweating.
- Rapid breathing.
- Restlessness.
- Shivering.
- Slow or fast pulse.
- Sudden jerky or shock-like movements.
- Tremor.
- The condition can become severe and may lead to a life-threatening situation.

Severe symptoms include,

- High fever.
- Losing consciousness.
- Seizures.
- Sudden swings in blood pressure and/or pulse.

(https://www.verywellmind.com › what-is-serotonin-syndrome-379651 accessed 7 February 2025).

Drugs that can cause serotonin syndrome include:

- Serotonin and norepinephrine reuptake inhibitors (SSRIs, SNRIs) such as citalopram, fluoxetine, fluvoxamine, paroxetine, sertraline, desvenlafaxine, duloxetine, venlafaxine.
- Monoamine oxidase inhibitors (MAOIs) such as isocarboxazid, phenelzine.
- Buspirone.
- Trazodone.
- Migraine treatments – almotriptan, eletriptan, rizatriptan.
- Pain medications such as fentanyl, hydrocodone, methadone, oxycodone, tramadol, tapentadol.
- Dextromethorphan – over the counter cough suppressant.
- Anti-nausea medications – metoclopramide, ondansetron.
- Lithium.
- Supplements - St John's wort, L-tryptophan, 5 hydroxy tryptophan (5 HTP).

Generally, MB is safe at levels less than 2 mg/kg, when given intravenously. Serotonin syndrome has been found to occur in doses of 5 mg/kg (Bistas & Sanghavi, 2023).

However, Schwiebert, Irving, and Gillman (2009) report on a case where a 1 mg/kg intravenous dose precipitated serotonin syndrome.

It is important to point out that nearly all the reported cases of serotonin syndrome were when MB was given intravenously during a surgical procedure (and the person was on an SSRI).

Schwiebert, Irving, and Gillman (2009) concluded *"We conclude that the use of MB by infusion in combination with other 5-hydroxytryptaminergic agents could lead to the ST [serotonin toxicity] syndrome as a result of MAO A inhibition."*

As mentioned above, nearly all case reports of serotonin syndrome have been associated with *intravenous* MB administration. Oral doses seem to be much less likely to cause serotonin syndrome. The issue is in rate of rise of MB levels. Intravenous MB has a rapid rise in blood levels while the oral dose has a much slower rate of rise. The intravenous route goes straight into the blood stream. With the oral route, the overall dose is less; metabolism starts in the stomach, there is the liver "first pass effect" before MB even enters the bloodstream.

However, there is one case report of a patient with major depressive disorder and generalised anxiety disorder, who was stable on venlafaxine, buspirone, bupropion and zolpidem. He was put on a medication after bladder surgery which contained MB 10 mgs per capsule. The standard dose was 1 capsule four times a day. This would mean he was taking up to 40 mgs of MB daily. He developed symptoms of increased anxiety, fidgetiness, insomnia, as well increased sweating, tremor, and mild elevations in blood pressure and body temperature, consistent with serotonin syndrome (Zuschlag, Warren, & Schultz, 2018).

Serotonin syndrome can happen with oral MB but is extremely rare but not impossible. Also note that the dose in the above case was relatively high – 40 mgs daily. I generally recommend lower doses.

Tariq et al. (2021) showed that a small dose of MB given during an endoscopic procedure is safe. They concluded that *"Serious AEs [adverse events] due to oral administration of MB are rare (n = 3, 0.16%). MB-related non-serious AEs are mild, self-limiting, and show a dose-related trend. These findings indicate that it is safe to use small amounts of MB as a food dye during swallowing examinations."*

As mentioned earlier, MB has MAO inhibiting (MAOI) activity. For this reason, there may be a concern that eating foods containing tyramine may be of concern. The concern is that MAO also metabolises tyramine and therefore MAOI reduces the metabolism of tyramine. Tyramine levels can rise and cause hypertension spikes that can be dangerous. Therefore, tyramine is best avoided while taking pharmaceutical MAOIs.

Foods high in tyramine:

- Aged meats.
- Cured/smoked meats – salami.
- Fermented foods – pickles, kim chi, sauerkraut.
- Aged, strong cheeses - cheddar, blue cheese, Swiss, parmesan, feta, camembert, gorgonzola, gruyère, provolone, and roquefort.
- Soybean products
- Soybean paste.
- Tofu.
- Soy sauce.
- Beer, stouts, porter, dark beers.
- Wine, robust red wines (white wine minimal).
- Sherry, vermouth, liqueurs.
- Dried/over-ripe fruits.
- Stored, or improperly stored foods can be high in tyramine. Fresh food is best.

You will be happy to know that chocolate is not high in tyramines!

Also note that many of these foods can combine, so a person on MAOI and drinking red wine and eating sauerkraut and lots of cheese may get into trouble.

Theoretically, MB, in conjunction with eating these foods could trigger a hypertension crisis reaction, the same as if on a pharmaceutical MAOI.

However, according to Gillman (2017), the level of tyramine is not as high as commonly thought. He explains that in the last decade, there have been changes in food production techniques which have reduced the level of tyramine in food. *"The main change has been the near-universal adoption of non-decarboxylating starter cultures, which do not produce any Tyr [tyramine]. Those are now used by almost all producers of cheeses, salamis, soy sauces, etc, and in consequence, modern diets have greatly reduced levels of Tyr."*

He concludes that *"... it is unlikely that injurious quantities [of tyramine] will be ingested."*

Note that the Gillman paper was discussing tyramine in relation to the use of MAOI pharmaceuticals. As MB has MAOI actions, the narrative is relevant.

A standard dose of MB, 3-5 mgs daily, is very unlikely to produce serotonin syndrome, BUT it would be best to avoid taking MB with an SSRI, though this may be difficult as there are so many people taking SSRIs!

Pulmonary hypertension

Another group of people who shouldn't take MB are those with pulmonary hypertension. In a letter to the editor, Hajj-Chahine, Jayle, and Corbi (2013) reiterated that one effect of MB is to reduce NO which *"can cause a significant increase in pulmonary arterial pressure, especially in patients with severe pulmonary hypertension and cause a detrimental effect on gas exchange."*

Not everyone can take MB.

Side effects

All medications can cause side effects, and MB is no exception.

Common side effects include:

- Gastrointestinal – nausea, upset stomach, vomiting, diarrhoea.
- Bladder irritation.
- Blue urine, blue stools. This is not dangerous, however, if the person is not warned, it may cause concern.
- More serious side effects include dizziness, fainting, high fever, anxiety, fast/irregular heartbeat –

this could indicate a possible **serotonin syndrome.**

- Pale blue skin can occur, as paradoxically, high doses of MB can cause a methaemoglobinaemia.
- Cardiovascular – increased BP and palpitations – not common.
- Central Nervous system – dizziness, headache, mental confusion (though this could be the start of serotonin syndrome).
- Fatigue.
- Fever.
- A rare serious side effect is chest pain – seek immediate medical attention.
- Also rarely, there can be an allergic reaction to MB, rash, itch, swelling, wheeze and difficult breathing. In severe cases there may be anaphylaxis. However, MB, in certain circumstances, can be used to treat anaphylaxis. *"We propose methylene blue as a safe treatment option for refractory anaphylaxis, whether with or without hypotension"* (Bauer, Vadas, & Kelly, 2013).
- Haemolytic anaemia if the person has a G6PD deficiency.

Large oral doses (greater than 30 mgs) of MB can affect the microbiome because of its antibiotic properties and may cause gut dysbiosis.

MB can interfere with pulse oximetry. This is especially so with large intravenous doses. Pulse oximetry is a method for monitoring blood oxygen saturation. Generally, the pulse oximeter is clipped onto a finger and peripheral oxygen saturation is measured.

"Intravenous dyes such as methylene blue or indocyanine green, sometimes used for surgical or diagnostic procedures, will color the serum in the blood and may interfere with the light absorption spectrum, resulting in falsely low readings" (Torp, Modi, Pollard, & Simon, 2023).

This is only relevant with intravenous MB injection during surgery. Smaller oral doses probably do not have this issue.

It is important to point out that these symptoms are dose dependant. Low doses are less likely to produce these symptoms.

Dosage is important.
High dose – intravenous – use once or twice – acute situation
Low dose – oral – regular use – chronic usage

LEGAL ASPECTS

The legal aspect can be complex. MB is classed as a Schedule 4 (S4) substance by the Therapeutics Goods Administration (TGA), which means that it is only legal for medicinal use if prescribed by a registered medical practitioner. Therefore, the sale of MB is a criminal offence. However, MB can be easily purchased on-line from many internet sites.

Purchasing MB for personal medical use without a prescription is illegal.

In Australia, the federal TGA classes MB as an S4, however, there are also different laws at the state level.

I live and practice in Tasmania, so I will only state the Tasmanian regulations.

"In Tasmania, under section 26 of the Poisons Act 1971 *(Tas), it is an offence to sell or supply medicinal substances without authorisation.*

The offence carries a maximum penalty of a fine of 10 penalty units. Medical practitioners, pharmacists, licensed chemists, dentists, authorised health professionals, veterinary surgeons, and authorised nurse practitioners acting within their lawful practice are permitted to sell or supply these substances. "

So, in Tasmania, as a registered medical practitioner, I can sell and supply this product.

For interstate readers, refer to the below website to review your local state laws. For overseas readers, I recommend you refer to your local laws.

(https://www.criminaldefencelawyers.com.au/blog/is-methylene-blue-legal-in-australia/ accessed 12 September 2025).

CONCLUSION

We have seen how MB can be used in the hospital situation, and throughout this book we have discussed how MB might be used outside of the hospital. An individual under the care of a doctor who understands and values the benefits of MB could support a patient wishing to try MB. This is especially so in situations where there is no cure, and where the mainstream/ conventional practitioners would prescribe a pharmaceutical approach, which, in many instances may be worse than the disease.

Pharmaceuticals are known for their unwanted side effects.

We have also discussed the benefits of MB in situations where the patient describes symptoms, yet rather than a diagnosis being given, a name is made up which simply describes the symptoms e.g. long COVID syndrome or chronic fatigue syndrome. The underlying pathophysiology in many cases is inflammation, and the reason for MB being beneficial in these instances is that it is known to be a simple, safe and inexpensive product that works well to combat inflammation and oxidation issues. It can get to the root cause of symptoms such as fatigue, brain fog, depression, anxiety and even pain.

The purpose of this book has been to present the reader with enough information about MB, a proven safe and very helpful treatment, so that they may make an informed decision about whether this may be right for them. Below is a summary of the attributes and benefits of MB.

It has an action on the mitochondria. Many diseases develop mitochondrial dysfunction, and MB can be used to improve mitochondrial function.

1. It can act as an antioxidant.
2. It has anti-inflammatory properties.
3. It has a monoamine oxidase inhibiting action, which can increase levels of serotonin, therefore, to treat depression.
4. It has antibacterial, antiviral, antimalarial, anti-cancer and antifungal activity.
5. It has nitric oxide synthase activity.
6. It has pain relieving properties.
7. As it is one of the few substances that can cross the blood brain barrier, it can reduce neuroinflammation, therefore can be used in neurodegenerative conditions.

Benefits of MB include:

1. Cognitive enhancement.
2. Anti-ageing properties.
3. Physical health benefits.
4. Memory and learning improvement.
5. Focus and concentration.
6. Neuroprotection.
7. Mitochondrial support.
8. Antioxidant effects.
9. Anti-inflammation.
10. Pain relief.
11. Cellular health.
12. Energy and metabolism boost.
13. Skin health.
14. Immune system support.

Given the benefits outlined above, MB can be considered in most chronic diseases, while, of course, being mindful of the precautions that have also been discussed.

Safe and effective dosages for those where MB is not contraindicated have been outlined in a number of places throughout the book.

As always, I recommend that MB be considered as a part of a wholistic approach to treatment. Diet, nutrition, supplements, herbs, exercise, good sleep, sunshine and stress reduction must always be considered as essential in any treatment protocol.

A lack of double-blind studies (which may never be done since MB is off patent and inexpensive) is not a reason to wait to incorporate this very useful product into the treatment regimens of patients who would most definitely benefit from it.

MB is a versatile compound that can be used to treat many diseases in many ways.

REFERENCES

Abahssain, H., Moukafih, B., Essangri, H., Mrabti, H., Meddah, B., Guessous, F., ...Errihani H. (2021). Methylene blue and ifosfamide-induced encephalopathy: Myth or reality? *J Oncol Pharm Pract, 27*(1), 143-149. doi: 10.1177/1078155220971843

Achan, J., Talisuna, A., Erhart, A., Yeka, A., Tibenderana, J., Baliraine, F., ... D'Alessandro U. (2011). Quinine, an old anti-malarial drug in a modern world: Role in the treatment of malaria. *Malar J, 10*, 144. doi: 10.1186/1475-2875-10-144

Aghahosseini, F., Arbabi-Kalati, F., Fashtami, L., Fateh, M., & Djavid, G. (2006). Treatment of oral lichen planus with photodynamic therapy mediated methylene blue: A case report. *Med Oral Patol Oral Cir Bucal, 11*(2), E126-9.

Ahn, H., Kang, S., Yoon, S., Ko, H., Kim, P., Hong, E., ... Lee G. (2017). Methylene blue inhibits NLRP3, NLRC4, AIM2, and non-canonical inflammasome activation. *Sci Rep, 7*(1), 12409. doi: 10.1038/s41598-017-12635-6

Alberdi, E., & Gómez, C. (2019). Efficiency of methylene blue-mediated photodynamic therapy vs intense pulsed light in the treatment of onychomycosis in the toenails. *Photodermatol Photoimmunol Photomed, 35*(2), 69-77. doi: 10.1111/phpp.12420

Alberdi, E., & Gómez, C. (2020). Successful treatment of Pityriasis Versicolor by photodynamic therapy mediated by methylene blue. *Photodermatol Photoimmunol Photomed, 36*(4), 308-312. doi: 10.1111/phpp.12555

Alda, M. (2019). Methylene blue in the treatment of neuropsychiatric disorders. *CNS Drugs, 33*(8), 719-725. doi: 10.1007/s40263-019-00641-3

Alda, M., McKinnon, M., Blagdon, R., Garnham, J., MacLellan, S., O'Donovan, C., … MacQueen, G. (2017). Methylene blue treatment for residual symptoms of bipolar disorder: Randomised crossover study. *Br J Psychiatry, 210*(1), 54-60. doi: 10.1192/bjp.bp.115.173930

Atamna, H., Nguyen, A., Schultz, C., Boyle, K., Newberry, J., Kato, H., & Ames, B. (2008). Methylene blue delays cellular senescence and enhances key mitochondrial biochemical pathways. *FASEB J, 22*(3), 703-12. doi: 10.1096/fj.07-9610com

Auchter, A., Williams, J., Barksdale, B., Monfils, M., & Gonzalez-Lima, F. (2014). Therapeutic benefits of methylene blue on cognitive impairment during chronic cerebral hypoperfusion. *J Alzheimers Dis, 42* Suppl 4, S525-35. doi: 10.3233/JAD-141527

Audet, J., Soucy, G., & Julien, J. (2012). Methylene blue administration fails to confer neuroprotection in two amyotrophic lateral sclerosis mouse models. *Neuroscience, 209*, 136-43. doi: 10.1016/j.neuroscience.2011.12.047

Azhough, R., Jalali, P., Dashti, M., Taher, S., & Aghajani, A. (2024). Intradermal methylene blue analgesic application in posthemorrhoidectomy pain management: A randomized controlled trial. *Front Surg, 11*, 1354328. doi: 10.3389/fsurg.2024.1354328

Baird, J. (2019). 8-Aminoquinoline therapy for latent malaria. *Clin Microbiol Rev, 32*(4), e00011-19. doi: 10.1128/CMR.00011-19

Balakumar, P., Venkatesan, K., Abdulla Khan, N., Raghavendra, N., Venugopal, V., Bharathi, D., & Fuloria, N. (2023). Mechanistic insights into the beneficial effects of curcumin on insulin resistance: Opportunities and challenges. *Drug Discov Today, 28*(7), 103627. doi: 10.1016/j.drudis.2023.103627

Bauer, C., Vadas, P., & Kelly, K. (2013). Methylene blue for the treatment of refractory anaphylaxis without hypotension. *Am J Emerg Med, 31*(1), 264.e3-5. doi: 10.1016/j.ajem.2012.03.036

Belotto, R., Chavantes, M., Tardivo, J., Euzébio Dos Santos, R., Fernandes, R., Horliana, A., ... Teixeira da Silva, D. (2017). Therapeutic comparison between treatments for vulvar lichen sclerosus: Study protocol of a randomized prospective and controlled trial. *BMC Womens Health, 17*(1), 61. doi: 10.1186/s12905-017-0414-y

Berthiaume, J., Hsiung, C., Austin, A., McBrayer, S., Depuydt, M., Chandler, M., ... Rosca, M. (2017). Methylene blue decreases mitochondrial lysine acetylation in the diabetic heart. *Mol Cell Biochem, 432*(1-2),7-24. doi: 10.1007/s11010-017-2993-1

Beshay, A., El Kahky, H., & Mohammad, G. (2023). Evaluation of daylight methylene blue photodynamic therapy in multiple recurrent molluscum contagiosum. *QJM: An International Journal of Medicine,* 116, Supplement_1, hcad069.212. doi: 10.1093/qjmed/hcad069.212

Bewick, J., & Pfleiderer, A. (2014). The value and role of low dose methylene blue in the surgical management of hyperparathyroidism. *Ann R Coll Surg Engl, 96*(7), 526-9. doi: 10.1308/003588414X13946184903883

Birch, A., & Boyce, W. (1976). Hypertension and decreased renal blood flow following methylene blue injection. *Anesth Analg, 55*(5), 674-6.

Birder, L. (2019). Pathophysiology of interstitial cystitis. *Int J Urol, 26 Suppl 1*, 12-15. doi: 10.1111/iju.13985

Bistas, E., & Sanghavi, D. (2025) *Methylene Blue*. [Updated 2023 Jun 26]. In: StatPearls [Internet]. Treasure Island (FL): StatPearls Publishing. Available from: https://www.ncbi.nlm.nih.gov/books/NBK557593/

Botros, M., Kesar, V., Seoud, T., Kesar, V Chimpiri, A., Sun, E., & Tzimas, D. (2017). Methylene blue dye for visual confirmation of enterocutaneous fistula. *American Journal of Gastroenterology 112*():p S1585.

Bountogo, M., Zoungrana, A., Coulibaly, B., Klose, C., Mansmann, U., Mockenhaupt, F., ... Müller O. (2010). Efficacy of methylene blue monotherapy in semi-immune adults with uncomplicated falciparum malaria: A controlled trial in Burkina Faso. *Trop Med Int Health, 15*(6), 713-7. doi: 10.1111/j.1365-3156.2010.02526.x

Bowornsathitchai, N., Thammahong, A., Shoosanglertwijit, J., Kitsongsermthon, J., Wititsuwannakul, J., Asawanonda, P., & Boontaveeyuwat, E. (2021). Methylene blue-mediated photodynamic therapy may be superior to 5% amorolfine nail lacquer for non-dermatophyte onychomycosis. *Photodermatol Photoimmunol Photomed, 37*(3), 183-191. doi: 10.1111/phpp.12624

Bruchey, A., & Gonzalez-Lima, F. (2008). Behavioral, physiological and biochemical hormetic responses to the autoxidizable dye methylene blue. *Am J Pharmacol Toxicol, 3*(1), 72-79. doi: 10.3844/ajptsp.2008.72.79

Cagno, V., Medaglia, C., Cerny, A., Cerny, T., Zwygart, A., Cerny, E., & Tapparel, C. (2021). Methylene blue has a potent antiviral activity against SARS-CoV-2 and H1N1 influenza virus in the absence of UV-activation in vitro. *Sci Rep, 11*(1), 14295. doi: 10.1038/s41598-021-92481-9

Canto, M., Setrakian, S., Willis, J., Chak, A., Petras, R., Powe, N., & Sivak, M. Jr. (2000). Methylene blue-directed biopsies improve detection of intestinal metaplasia and dysplasia in Barrett's esophagus. *Gastrointest Endosc, 51*(5), 560-8. doi: 10.1016/s0016-5107(00)70290-2

Carvalho, A., Gonçalves, N., Teixeira, P., Goulart, A., & Leão, P. (2024). The impact of methylene blue in colorectal cancer: Systematic review and meta-analysis study. *Surg Oncol, 53*, 102046. doi: 10.1016/j.suronc.2024.102046

Cavaliere, P., Torrent, J., Prigent, S., Granata, V., Pauwels, K., Pastore, A., ... Zagari, A. (2013). Binding of methylene blue to a surface cleft inhibits the oligomerization and fibrillization of prion protein. *Biochim Biophys Acta, 1832*(1), 20-8. doi: 10.1016/j.bbadis.2012.09.005

Cawein, M., Behlen, C. 2nd., Lappat, E., & Cohn, J. (1964). Hereditary diaphorase deficiency and methemoglobinemia. *Arch Intern Med, 113*, 578-85. doi: 10.1001/archinte.1964.00280100086014

Cesar, G., Winyk, A., Sluchensci Dos Santos, F., Queiroz, E., Soares, K., Caetano, W., & Tominaga, T. (2022). Treatment of chronic wounds with methylene blue photodynamic therapy: A case report. *Photodiagnosis Photodyn Ther, 39*, 103016. doi: 10.1016/j.pdpdt.2022.103016

Chang, T., Fiumara, N., & Weinstein, L. (1975). Genital herpes: Treatment with methylene blue and light exposure. *Int J Dermatol, 14*(1), 69-71. doi: 10.1111/j.1365-4362.1975.tb00084.x

Chang, T., & Weinstein, L. (1975). Eczema herpeticum. Treatment with methylene blue and light. *Arch Dermatol, 111*(9), 1174-5. doi: 10.1001/archderm.111.9.1174

Chuang, S., Papp, H., Kuczmog, A., Eells, R., Condor Capcha, J., Shehadeh, L., ... Buchwald, P. (2022). Methylene blue is a nonspecific protein-protein interaction inhibitor with potential for repurposing as an antiviral for COVID-19. *Pharmaceuticals (Basel), 15*(5), 621. doi: 10.3390/ph15050621

Cirrincione, A., Pellegrini, A., Dominy, J., Benjamin, M., Utkina-Sosunova, I., Lotti, F., ... Rieger, S. (2020). Paclitaxel-induced peripheral neuropathy is caused by epidermal ROS and mitochondrial damage through conserved MMP-13 activation. *Sci Rep, 10*(1), 3970. doi: 10.1038/s41598-020-60990-8

Correia, J., Rodrigues, J., Pimenta, S., Dong, T., & Yang, Z. (2021). Photodynamic therapy review: Principles, photosensitizers, applications, and future directions. *Pharmaceutics, 13*(9), 1332. doi: 10.3390/pharmaceutics13091332

Coulibaly, B., Zoungrana, A., Mockenhaupt, F., Schirmer, R., Klose, C., Mansmann, U., … Müller, O. (2009). Strong gametocytocidal effect of methylene blue-based combination therapy against falciparum malaria: A randomised controlled trial. *PLoS One, 4*(5), e5318. doi: 10.1371/journal.pone.0005318

Cui, J., Zhang, J., Zhang, Y., & Ma, Z. (2016). [Efficacy of intracutaneous methylene blue injection for moderate to severe acute thoracic herpes zoster pain and prevention of postherpetic neuralgia in elderly patients]. *Nan Fang Yi Ke Da Xue Xue Bao, 36*(10), 1377-1381. Chinese.

da Silva, A., Barreto de Abreu, P., Geraldes, D., & Nascimento, L. (2021). Hydroxychloroquine: Pharmacological, physicochemical aspects and activity enhancement through experimental formulations. *Journal of Drug Delivery Science and Technology, 63*, 102512. doi:10.1016/j.jddst.2021.102512

Dabholkar, N., Gorantla, S., Dubey, S., Alexander, A., Taliyan, R., & Singhvi, G. (2021). Repurposing methylene blue in the management of COVID-19: Mechanistic aspects and clinical investigations. *Biomed Pharmacother, 142*, 112023. doi: 10.1016/j.biopha.2021.112023

Delport, A., Harvey, B., Petzer, A., & Petzer, J. (2017). Methylene blue and its analogues as antidepressant compounds. *Metab Brain Dis, 32*(5), 1357-1382. doi: 10.1007/s11011-017-0081-6

Deng, M., Huang, H., Ma, Y., Zhou, Y., Chen, Q., & Xie, P. (2021). Intradiskal injection of methylene blue for discogenic back pain: A meta-analysis of randomized controlled trials. *J Neurol Surg A Cent Eur Neurosurg, 82*(2), 161-165. doi: 10.1055/s-0040-1721015

Deng, Y., Yang, Y., Zhu, F., Liu, W., Chen, J., & Xu, G. (2025). Analgesic efficacy and safety of methylene blue combined with cocktail for periarticular infiltration following total knee arthroplasty: A prospective, randomized, controlled study. *Perioper Med (Lond), 14*(1), 9. doi: 10.1186/s13741-025-00493-0

Deutsch, S., Rosse, R., Schwartz, B., Fay-McCarthy, M., Rosenberg, P., & Fearing K. (1997). Methylene blue adjuvant therapy of schizophrenia. *Clin Neuropharmacol, 20*(4), 357-63. doi: 10.1097/00002826-199708000-00008

Doll, D., Novotny, A., Rothe, R., Kristiansen, J., Wietelmann, K., Boulesteix, A., ... Petersen, S. (2008). Methylene Blue halves the long-term recurrence rate in acute pilonidal sinus disease. *Int J Colorectal Dis, 23*(2), 181-7. doi: 10.1007/s00384-007-0393-9

Dondas, A., Luca, A., Alexa, T., Grigoras, V., Mungiu, O., & Bohotin, C. (2013). Repeated methylene blue administration produces analgesia in experimental pain. *J Headache Pain 14* (Suppl 1), P86. doi: 10.1186/1129-2377-14-S1-P86

Dorafshar, A., Gitman, M., Henry, G., Agarwal, S., & Gottlieb, L. (2010). Guided surgical debridement: Staining tissues with methylene blue. *J Burn Care Res, 31*(5), 791-4. doi: 10.1097/BCR.0b013e3181eed1d6

Duicu, O., Privistirescu, A., Wolf, A., Petruş, A., Dănilă, M., Raţiu, C., ... Sturza, A. (2017). Methylene blue improves mitochondrial respiration and decreases oxidative stress in a substrate-dependent manner in diabetic rat hearts. *Can J Physiol Pharmacol, 95*(11), 1376-1382. doi: 10.1139/cjpp-2017-0074

Durgut, H. (2018). Methylene blue provides an efficient resection for the treatment of pilonidal sinus disease. *Selcuk Med J, 34*(1), 6-10. doi: 10.30733/std.2018.01013

Dwyer, B., & Katz, D. (2018). Postconcussion syndrome. *Handb Clin Neurol, 158*, 163-178. doi: 10.1016/B978-0-444-63954-7.00017-3

Emadi, E., Hamidi Alamdari, D., Attaran, D., & Attaran, S. (2024). Application of methylene blue for the prevention and treatment of COVID-19: A narrative review. *Iran J Basic Med Sci, 27*(7), 780-792. doi: 10.22038/IJBMS.2024.71871.15617

Eroğlu, L., & Cağlayan, B. (1997). Anxiolytic and antidepressant properties of methylene blue in animal models. *Pharmacol Res, 36*(5), 381-5. doi: 10.1006/phrs.1997.0245

Esser, N., Paquot, N., & Scheen, A. (2015). Anti-inflammatory agents to treat or prevent type 2 diabetes, metabolic syndrome and cardiovascular disease. *Expert Opin Investig Drugs, 24*(3), 283-307. doi: 10.1517/13543784.2015.974804

Fadel, M., Salah, M., Samy, N., &Mona, S. (2009). Liposomal methylene blue hydrogel for selective photodynamic therapy of acne vulgaris. *J Drugs Dermatol, 8*(11), 983-90.

Fathy, G., Asaad, M., & Rasheed, H. (2017). Daylight photodynamic therapy with methylene blue in plane warts: A randomized double-blind placebo-controlled study. *Photodermatol Photoimmunol Photomed, 33*(4), 185-192. doi: 10.1111/phpp.12291

Feng, J., Weitner, M., Shi, W., Zhang, S., Sullivan, D., & Zhang, Y. (2015). Identification of additional anti-persister activity against Borrelia burgdorferi from an FDA drug library. *Antibiotics (Basel), 4*(3), 397-410. doi: 10.3390/antibiotics4030397

Filler, K., Lyon, D., Bennett, J., McCain, N., Elswick, R., Lukkahatai, N., & Saligan, L. (2014). Association of mitochondrial dysfunction and fatigue: A review of the literature. *BBA Clin, 1*, 12-23. doi: 10.1016/j.bbacli.2014.04.001

Frye, R. (2020). Mitochondrial dysfunction in autism spectrum disorder: Unique abnormalities and targeted treatments. *Semin Pediatr Neurol, 35*, 100829. doi: 10.1016/j.spen.2020.100829

Gama, C., Pombo, M., Nunes, C., Gama, G., Mezitis,S., Suchmacher Neto, M., ... Darrigo Junior, L. (2020). Treatment of recurrent urinary tract infection symptoms with urinary antiseptics containing methenamine and methylene blue: Analysis of etiology and treatment outcomes. *Res Rep Urol, 12*, 639-649. doi: 10.2147/RRU.S279060

Geiger, J. (1933). Methylene blue solution in the treatment of carbon monoxide poisoning. *JAMA, 100*(14). 1103-1104. doi:10.1001/jama.1933.27420140001008a

Gendrot, M., Andreani, J., Duflot, I., Boxberger, M., Le Bideau, M., Mosnier, J., ... Pradines, B. (2020).

Methylene blue inhibits replication of SARS-CoV-2 in vitro. *Int J Antimicrob Agents, 56*(6), 106202. doi: 10.1016/j.ijantimicag.2020.106202

Genrikhs, E., Stelmashook, E., Voronkov, D., Novikova, S., Alexandrova, O., Gulyaev, M., & Isaev, N. (2020). The delayed neuroprotective effect of methylene blue in experimental rat brain trauma. *Antioxidants (Basel), 9*(5), 377. doi: 10.3390/antiox9050377

Ghanizadeh, A., Berk, M., Farrashbandi, H., Alavi Shoushtari, A., & Villagonzalo, K. (2013). Targeting the mitochondrial electron transport chain in autism, a systematic review and synthesis of a novel therapeutic approach. *Mitochondrion, 13*(5), 515-9. doi: 10.1016/j.mito.2012.10.001

Gillman, K. (2017). "Much ado about nothing": Monoamine oxidase inhibitors, drug interactions, and dietary tyramine. *CNS Spectr, 22*(5), 385-387. doi: 10.1017/S1092852916000651

Gonzalez-Lima, F., & Auchter, A. (2015). Protection against neurodegeneration with low-dose methylene blue and near-infrared light. *Front Cell Neurosci, 9*, 179. doi: 10.3389/fncel.2015.00179

Goyal, A. (2018). New technologies for sentinel lymph node detection. *Breast Care (Basel), 13*(5), 349-353. doi: 10.1159/000492436

Grande, M., Miyake, A., Nagamine, M., Leite, J., da Fonseca, I., Massoco, C., & Dagli, M. (2022). Methylene blue and photodynamic therapy for melanomas: Inducing different rates of cell death (necrosis and apoptosis) in B16-F10 melanoma cells according to methylene blue concentration and energy dose. *Photodiagnosis Photodyn Ther, 37,* 102635. doi: 10.1016/j.pdpdt.2021.102635

Grauman Neander, N., Loner, C., & Rotoli, J. (2018). The acute treatment of methemoglobinemia in pregnancy. *J Emerg Med, 54*(5), 685-689. doi: 10.1016/j.jemermed.2018.01.038

Guo, X., Ding, W., Liu, L., & Yang, S. (2019). Intradiscal methylene blue injection for discogenic low back pain: A meta-analysis. *Pain Pract, 19*(1), 118-129. doi: 10.1111/papr.12725

Gupta, G., Radhakrishna, M., Chankowsky, J., & Asenjo, J. (2012). Methylene blue in the treatment of discogenic low back pain. *Pain Physician, 15*(4), 333-8.

Hajj-Chahine, J., Jayle, C., & Corbi, P. (2013). Methylene blue in patients with severe pulmonary hypertension. *J Thorac Cardiovasc Surg, 145*(3), 898. doi: 10.1016/j.jtcvs.2012.11.091

Hamilton, C., El Khoury, H., Hamilton, D., Nicklason, F., & Mitrofanis, J. (2019). "Buckets": Early observations on the use of red and infrared light helmets in Parkinson's disease patients. *Photobiomodul Photomed Laser Surg, 37*(10), 615-622. doi: 10.1089/photob.2019.4663

Hanash, K., Al Zahrani, H., Mokhtar, A., & Aslam, M. (2003). Retrograde vaginal methylene blue injection for localization of complex urinary fistulas. *J Endourol, 17*(10), 941-3. doi: 10.1089/089277903772036334

Hanzlik, P. (1933). Methylene blue as antidote for cyanide poisoning. *JAMA, 100*(5), 357. doi: 10.1001/jama.1933.02740050053028

Haouzi, P., Gueguinou, M., Sonobe, T., Judenherc-Haouzi, A., Tubbs, N., Trebak, M., ... Bouillaud, F. (2018). Revisiting the physiological effects of methylene blue as a treatment of cyanide intoxication. *Clin Toxicol (Phila), 56*(9), 828-840. doi: 10.1080/15563650.2018.1429615

Haouzi, P., McCann, M., Wang, J., Zhang, X., Song, J., Sariyer, I., ... Cheung, J. (2020). Antidotal effects of methylene blue against cyanide neurological toxicity: In vivo and in vitro studies. *Ann N Y Acad Sci, 1479*(1), 108-121. doi: 10.1111/nyas.14353

Hashmi, M., Ahmed, R., Mahmoud, S., Ahmed, K., Bushra, N., Ahmed, A., ... Abdelrahman, N. (2023). Exploring methylene blue and its derivatives in Alzheimer's treatment: A comprehensive review of randomized control trials. *Cureus, 15*(10), e46732. doi: 10.7759/cureus.46732

Howland, R. (2016). Methylene blue: The long and winding road from stain to brain: Part 1. *J Psychosoc Nurs Ment Health Serv, 54*(9), 21-4. doi: 10.3928/02793695-20160818-01

Howland, R. (2016). Methylene blue: The long and winding road from stain to brain: Part 2. *J Psychosoc Nurs Ment Health Serv. 54*(10), 21-26. doi: 10.3928/02793695-20160920-04

Hübler, J., Szántó, A., & Könyves, K. (2003). Methylene blue as a means of treatment for priapism caused by intracavernous injection to combat erectile dysfunction. *Int Urol Nephrol, 35*(4), 519-21. doi: 10.1023/b:urol.0000025617.97048.ae

Ibarra-Estrada, M., Kattan, E., Aguilera-González, P., Sandoval-Plascencia, L., Rico-Jauregui, U., Gómez-Partida, C., ... Hernández, G. (2023). Early adjunctive methylene blue in patients with septic shock: A randomized controlled trial. *Crit Care, 27*(1), 110. doi: 10.1186/s13054-023-04397-7

Isaev, N., Genrikhs, E., & Stelmashook, E. (2024). Methylene blue and its potential in the treatment of traumatic brain injury, brain ischemia, and Alzheimer's disease. *Rev Neurosci, 35*(5), 585-595. doi: 10.1515/revneuro-2024-0007

Kallewaard, J., Wintraecken, V., Geurts, J., Willems, P., van Santbrink, H., Terwiel, C., ... van Kuijk, S. (2019). A multicenter randomized controlled trial on the efficacy of intradiscal methylene blue injection for chronic discogenic low back pain: The IMBI study. *Pain, 160*(4), 945-953. doi: 10.1097/j.pain.0000000000001475

Kanjwal, K., Karabin, B., Kanjwal, Y., Saeed, B., & Grubb, B. (2010). Autonomic dysfunction presenting as orthostatic intolerance in patients suffering from mitochondrial cytopathy. *Clin Cardiol, 33*(10), 626-629. doi: 10.1002/clc.20805

Kaura, A., Shukla, R., Lamyman, A., Almeyda, R., Draper, M., Martinez-Devesa, P., & Qureishi, A. (2020). Photodynamic therapy as a new treatment for chronic rhinosinusitis: A systematic review. *Turk Arch Otorhinolaryngol, 58*(4), 254-267. doi: 10.5152/tao.2020.5218

Kawamoto, H., Watanabe, H., Yajin, K., & Kouro, O. (1999). Effects of methylene blue on human nasal allergy. *Practica oto-rhino-laryngologica, 1999*, 9-13.

Kearns, M., & Tangpricha, V. (2014). The role of vitamin D in tuberculosis. *J Clin Transl Endocrinol, 1*(4), 167-169. doi: 10.1016/j.jcte.2014.08.002

Khan, I., Saeed, K., Zekker, I., Zhang, B., Hendi, A. H., Ahmad, A., ... Khan, I. (2022). Review on methylene blue: Its properties, uses, toxicity and photodegradation. *Water, 14*(2), 242. https://doi.org/10.3390/w14020242

Kim, J., Kim, D., & Lee, Y. (2019). Long-term followup of intradermal injection of methylene blue for intractable, idiopathic pruritus ani. *Tech Coloproctol, 23*(2), 143-149. doi: 10.1007/s10151-019-01934-x

Kraus, R., Grof, P., Arana, G., Workman, R., Harvey, K., & Hux, M. (1987). Methylene blue: A reliable and practical marker for validating compliance on the DST. *J Clin Psychiatry, 48*(6), 224-9.

Kwak, S., Park, K., Lee, K., & Lee, H. (2010). Mitochondrial metabolism and diabetes. *J Diabetes Investig, 1*(5), 161-9. doi: 10.1111/j.2040-1124.2010.00047.x

Lambden, S., Creagh-Brown, B., Hunt, J., Summers, C., & Forni, L. (2018). Definitions and pathophysiology of vasoplegic shock. *Crit Care, 22*(1), 174. doi: 10.1186/s13054-018-2102-1

Lamptey, R., Chaulagain, B., Trivedi, R., Gothwal, A., Layek, B., & Singh, J. (2022). A review of the common neurodegenerative disorders: Current therapeutic approaches and the potential role of nanotherapeutics. *Int J Mol Sci, 23*(3), 1851. doi: 10.3390/ijms23031851

Le, M., Wuertz, B., Biel, M., Thompson, R., & Ondrey F. (2022). Effects of methylene blue photodynamic therapy on oral carcinoma and leukoplakia cells. *Laryngoscope Investig Otolaryngol, 7*(4), 982-987. doi: 10.1002/lio2.772

Lecor, P., Touré, B., Moreau, N., Braud, A., Dieb, W., & Boucher, Y. (2020). Could methylene blue be used to manage burning mouth syndrome? A pilot case series. *J Oral Med Oral Surg, 26*:35. Doi: 10.1051/mbcb/2020032

Lee, S., & Han, H. (2021). Methylene blue application to lessen pain: Its analgesic effect and mechanism. *Front Neurosci, 15*, 663650. doi: 10.3389/fnins.2021.663650

Lee, S., Moon, S., Park, J., Suh, H., & Han, H. (2021). Methylene blue induces an analgesic effect by significantly decreasing neural firing rates and improves pain behaviors in rats. *Biochem Biophys Res Commun, 541*, 36-42. doi: 10.1016/j.bbrc.2021.01.008

Lessey, B., Higdon, H.3rd., Miller, S., & Price, T. (2012). Intraoperative detection of subtle endometriosis: A novel paradigm for detection and treatment of pelvic pain associated with the loss of peritoneal integrity. *J Vis Exp. 2012*, (70), 4313. doi: 10.3791/4313

Levin, R., Degrange, M., Bruno, G., Del Mazo, C., Taborda, D., Griotti, J., & Boullon, F. (2004). Methylene blue reduces mortality and morbidity in vasoplegic patients after cardiac surgery. *Ann Thorac Surg, 77*(2), 496-9. doi: 10.1016/S0003-4975(03)01510-8

Li, J., Chen, X., Qi, M., & Li, Y. (2018). Sentinel lymph node biopsy mapped with methylene blue dye alone in patients with breast cancer: A systematic review and meta-analysis. *PLoS One, 13*(9), e0204364. doi: 10.1371/journal.pone.0204364

Li, J., Wang, R., Xu, J., Sun, K., Jiang, H., Sun, Z., … Shi, D. (2022). Methylene blue prevents osteoarthritis progression and relieves pain in rats via upregulation of Nrf2/PRDX1. *Acta Pharmacol Sin, 43*(2), 417-428. doi: 10.1038/s41401-021-00646-z

Li, T., Feng, J., Xiao, S., Shi, W., Sullivan, D., & Zhang, Y. (2019). Identification of FDA-approved drugs with activity against stationary phase *Bartonella henselae*. *Antibiotics (Basel), 8*(2), 50. doi: 10.3390/antibiotics8020050

Li, Y., & Ying, W. (2023). Methylene blue reduces the serum levels of interleukin-6 and inhibits STAT3 activation in the brain and the skin of lipopolysaccharide-administered mice. *Front Immunol, 14*, 1181932. doi: 10.3389/fimmu.2023.1181932

Li, Z., Lang, Y., Sakamuru, S., Samrat, S., Trudeau, N., Kuo, L., … Li, H. (2020). Methylene blue is a potent and broad-spectrum inhibitor against Zika virus *in vitro* and *in vivo*. *Emerg Microbes Infect, 209*(1), 2404-2416. doi: 10.1080/22221751.2020.1838954

Lin, A., Poteet, E., Du, F., Gourav, R., Liu, R., Wen, Y., ... Duong, T. (2012). Methylene blue as a cerebral metabolic and hemodynamic enhancer. *PLoS One, 7*(10), e46585. doi: 10.1371/journal.pone.0046585

Liu, Y., Wang, M., Xiong, M., Zhang, X., & Fang, M. (2020). Intravenous administration of vitamin C in the treatment of herpes zoster-associated pain: Two case reports and literature review. *Pain Res Manag, 2020*, 8857287. doi: 10.1155/2020/8857287

Lobascio, P., Tomasicchio, G., Cassetta, N., Altomare, D., Gallo, G., Pezzolla, A., & Laforgia, R. (2025). The use of a methylene blue and glyceryl trinitrate-based cream for the treatment of chronic anal fissures: A phase II randomized pilot trial from a referral coloproctological unit. *Tech Coloproctol, 29*(1), 39. doi: 10.1007/s10151-024-03029-8

Lu, G., Nagbanshi, M., Goldau, N., Mendes Jorge, M., Meissner, P., Jahn, A., ... Müller, O. (2018). Efficacy and safety of methylene blue in the treatment of malaria: A systematic review. *BMC Med, 16*(1), 59. doi: 10.1186/s12916-018-1045-3

Lu, Q, Tucker, D., Dong, Y., Zhao, N., & Zhang, Q. (2016). Neuroprotective and functional improvement effects of methylene blue in global cerebral ischemia.

Mol Neurobiol, 53(8), 5344-55. doi: 10.1007/s12035-015-9455-0

Martínez Portillo, F., Hoang-Boehm, J., Weiss, J., Alken, P., & Jünemann, K. (2001). Methylene blue as a successful treatment alternative for pharmacologically induced priapism. *Eur Urol, 39*(1), 20-3. doi: 10.1159/000052407

Mattson, M. (2007). Hormesis defined. *Ageing Res Rev, 7*(1), 1-7. doi: 10.1016/j.arr.2007.08.007

McEnerney, J., & McEnerney, L. (1983) Unfavorable neonatal outcome after intraamniotic injection of methylene blue. *Obstet Gynecol, 61*(3 Suppl), 35S-37S.

McGill Percy, K., Liu, Z., & Qi, X. (2025). Mitochondrial dysfunction in Alzheimer's disease: Guiding the path to targeted therapies. *Neurotherapeutics, 22*(3), e00525. doi: 10.1016/j.neurot.2025.e00525

Medina, D., Caccamo, A., & Oddo, S. (2011). Methylene blue reduces aβ levels and rescues early cognitive deficit by increasing proteasome activity. *Brain Pathol, 21*(2), 140-9. doi: 10.1111/j.1750-3639.2010.00430.x

Mehaffey, J., Johnston, L., Hawkins, R., Charles, E., Yarboro, L., Kern, J., … Ghanta, R. (2017). Methylene blue for vasoplegic syndrome after cardiac operation: Early administration improves survival. *Ann Thorac*

Surg, 104(1), 36-41. doi: 10.1016/j.atho-racsur.2017.02.057

Miller, L., Rojas-Jaimes, J., Low, L., & Corbellini, G. (2022). What historical records teach us about the discovery of quinine. *Am J Trop Med Hyg, 108*(1), 7-11. doi: 10.4269/ajtmh.22-0404

Miralles, L., López-Bas, R., Díaz-Alejo, C., & Roldan, C. (2024). Methylene blue, a unique topical analgesic: A case report. *J Palliat Med, 27*(10), 1425-1428. doi: 10.1089/jpm.2024.0033

Molnar, T., Lehoczki, A., Fekete, M., Varnai, R., Zavori, L., Erdo-Bonyar, S., ... Ezer, E. (2024). Mitochondrial dysfunction in long COVID: Mechanisms, consequences, and potential therapeutic approaches. *Geroscience, 46*(5), 5267-5286. doi: 10.1007/s11357-024-01165-5

Müller, O., Mockenhaupt, F., Marks, B., Meissner, P., Coulibaly, B., Kuhnert, R., ... Mansmann, U. (2013). Haemolysis risk in methylene blue treatment of G6PD-sufficient and G6PD-deficient West-African children with uncomplicated falciparum malaria: A synopsis of four RCTs. *Pharmacoepidemiol Drug Saf, 22*(4), 376-85. doi: 10.1002/pds.3370

Myhill, S., Booth, N., & McLaren-Howard, J. (2009). Chronic fatigue syndrome and mitochondrial dysfunction. *Int J Clin Exp Med, 2*(1), 1-16.

Nasim,F., Sakata, K., Schiavo, D., Nelson, D., Kern, R., & Mullon, J. (2017). Localizing bronchopleural fistula with methylene blue. *Chest, 152*(4), A881.

Naylor, G., Smith, A., & Connelly, P. (1987). A controlled trial of methylene blue in severe depressive illness. *Biol Psychiatry, 22*(5), 657-9. Doi: 10.1016/0006-3223(87)90194-6

Neagoe, O., Ionica, M., & Mazilu, O. (2018). Use of methylene blue in the prevention of recurrent intra-abdominal postoperative adhesions. *J Int Med Res, 46*(1), 504-510. doi: 10.1177/0300060517727694

Ng Ying Kin, S., Wei, M., Arachchi, A., & Bolshinsky, V. (2021). Retrograde injection of methylene blue as a technique for identification of obscure colonic fistulae. *ANZ J Surg, 91*(5), E353-E354. doi: 10.1111/ans.16377

Niyazov, D., Kahler, S., & Frye, R. (2016). Primary mitochondrial disease and secondary mitochondrial dysfunction: Importance of distinction for diagnosis and treatment. *Mol Syndromol, 7*(3), 122-37. doi: 10.1159/000446586

Oktay, S., Onat, F., Karahan, F., Alican, I., Ozkutlu, U., & Yegen, B. (1993). Effect of methylene blue on blood pressure in rats. *Pharmacology, 46*(4), 206-10. doi: 10.1159/000139047

Ommati, M., Azarpira, N., Gozashtegan, V., Khodaei, F., Niknahad, H., & Heidari, R. (2020). Methylene blue treatment enhances mitochondrial function and locomotor activity in a C57BL/6 mouse model of multiple sclerosis. *Trends in Pharmaceutical Sciences, 6*(1), 29-42. doi:10.30476/TIPS2020.85962.1044

Özdemir, A., Mayir, B., Demirbakan, K., & Oygür, N. (2014). Efficacy of methylene blue in sentinel lymph node biopsy for early breast cancer. *J Breast Health, 10*(2), 88-91. doi: 10.5152/tjbh.2014.1914

Özdemir, Ö., Kasımoğlu, G., Bak, A., Sütlüoğlu, H., & Savaşan, S. (2024). Mast cell activation syndrome: An up-to-date review of literature. *World J Clin Pediatr, 13*(2), 92813. doi: 10.5409/wjcp.v13.i2.92813

Ozkul, O., Ozkul, B., & Erbas, O. (2022). The investigation of ameliorating effect of methylene blue on cisplatin-induced neurotoxicity in female rats. *Journal of Clinical and Experimental Investigations, 13*(1), em00789. doi: 10.29333/jcei/11555

Pelgrims, J., De Vos, F., Van den Brande, J., Schrijvers, D., Prové, A., & Vermorken, J. (2000). Methylene blue in the treatment and prevention of ifosfamide-induced encephalopathy: Report of 12 cases and a review of the literature. *Br J Cancer, 82*(2), 291-4. doi: 10.1054/bjoc.1999.0917

Peng, B., Pang, X., Wu, Y., Zhao, C., & Song, X. (2010). A randomized placebo-controlled trial of intra-discal methylene blue injection for the treatment of chronic discogenic low back pain. *Pain, 149*(1), 124-129. doi: 10.1016/j.pain.2010.01.021

Polat, E., & Kang, K. (2021). Natural photosensitizers in antimicrobial photodynamic therapy. *Biomedicines, 9*(6), 584. doi: 10.3390/biomedicines9060584

Pominova, D., Ryabova, A., Skobeltsin, A., Markova, I., Linkov, K., & Romanishkin, I. (2024). The use of methylene blue to control the tumor oxygenation level. *Photodiagnosis Photodyn Ther, 46*, 104047. doi: 10.1016/j.pdpdt.2024.104047

Prasun, P. (2020). Mitochondrial dysfunction in meta-bolic syndrome. *Biochim Biophys Acta Mol Basis Dis, 1866*(10), 165838. doi: 10.1016/j.bbadis.2020.165838

Privistirescu, A., Sima, A., Duicu, O., Timar, R., Roşca, M., Sturza, A., & Muntean, D. (2018). Methylene blue alleviates endothelial dysfunction and reduces oxidative stress in aortas from diabetic rats. *Can J Physiol Pharmacol, 96*(10), 1012-1016. doi: 10.1139/cjpp-2018-0119

Ragunath, K., Krasner, N., Raman, V., Haqqani, M., & Cheung W. (2003). A randomized, prospective cross-over trial comparing methylene blue-directed biopsy and conventional random biopsy for detecting intestinal metaplasia and dysplasia in Barrett's esophagus. *Endos-copy, 35*(12), 998-1003. doi: 10.1055/s-2003-44599

Ramsay, R., Dunford, C., & Gillman, P. (2007). Methylene blue and serotonin toxicity: Inhibition of monoamine oxidase A (MAO A) confirms a theoretical prediction. *Br J Pharmacol. 152*(6), 946-51. doi: 10.1038/sj.bjp.0707430

Reddy, P., Lent-Schochet, D., Ramakrishnan, N., McLaughlin, M., & Jialal, I. (2019). Metabolic syndrome is an inflammatory disorder: A conspiracy between adipose tissue and phagocytes. *Clin Chim Acta, 496*, 35-44. doi: 10.1016/j.cca.2019.06.019

Rengelshausen, J., Burhenne, J., Fröhlich, M., Tayrouz, Y., Singh, S., Riedel, K., … Walter-Sack, I. (2004). Pharmacokinetic interaction of chloroquine and methylene blue combination against malaria. *Eur J Clin Pharmacol, 60*(10), 709-15. doi: 10.1007/s00228-004-0818-0

Rodriguez, P., Zhou, W., Barrett, D., Altmeyer, W., Gutierrez, J., Li, J., … Duong, T. (2016). Multimodal randomized functional MR imaging of the effects of methylene blue in the human brain. *Radiology, 281*(2), 516-526. doi: 10.1148/radiol.2016152893

Roldan, C., Rosenthal, D., Koyyalagunta, D., Feng, L., & Warner, K. (2023). Methylene blue for the treatment of radiation-induced oral mucositis during head and neck cancer treatment: An uncontrolled cohort. *Cancers (Basel), 15*(15),3994. doi: 10.3390/cancers15153994

Rosenkranz, S., Shaposhnykov, A., Träger, S., Engler, J., Witte, M., Roth, V., ... Friese, M. (2021). Enhancing mitochondrial activity in neurons protects against neurodegeneration in a mouse model of multiple sclerosis. *Elife, 10*, e61798. doi: 10.7554/eLife.61798

Sadaksharam, J., Nayaki, K., & Selvam, N. (2012). Treatment of oral lichen planus with methylene blue mediated photodynamic therapy--a clinical study. *Photodermatol Photoimmunol Photomed, 28*(2), 97-101. doi: 10.1111/j.1600-0781.2012.00647.x

Saklayen, M. (2018). The global epidemic of the metabolic syndrome. *Curr Hypertens Rep, 20*(2), 12. doi: 10.1007/s11906-018-0812-z

Salah, M., Samy, N., & Fadel, M. (2009). Methylene blue mediated photodynamic therapy for resistant plaque psoriasis. *J Drugs Dermatol, 8*(1), 42-9.

Sanchala, D., Bhatt, L., Pethe, P., Shelat, R., & Kulkarni, Y. (2018). Anticancer activity of methylene blue via inhibition of heat shock protein 70. *Biomed Pharmacother, 107*, 1037-1045. doi: 10.1016/j.biopha.2018.08.095

Schencking, M., Vollbracht, C., Weiss, G., Lebert, J., Biller, A., Goyvaerts, B., & Kraft, K. (2012).

Intravenous vitamin C in the treatment of shingles: Results of a multicenter prospective cohort study. *Med Sci Monit, 18*(4), CR215-24. doi: 10.12659/msm.882621

Schirmer,H., Adler, H., Pickhardt, M., & Mandelkow, E. (2011). "Lest we forget you--methylene blue...". *Neurobiol Aging, 32*(12), 2325.e7-16. doi: 10.1016/j.neurobiolaging.2010.12.01

Schwiebert, C., Irving, C., & Gillman, P. (2009). Small doses of methylene blue, previously considered safe, can precipitate serotonin toxicity. *Anaesthesia, 64*(8), 924. doi: 10.1111/j.1365-2044.2009.06029.x

Scigliano, G., & Scigliano, G. (2021). Methylene blue in covid-19. *Med Hypotheses, 146*, 110455. doi: 10.1016/j.mehy.2020.110455

Şen Tanrıkulu, C., Tanrıkulu, Y., Kılınç, F., Bahadır, B., Can, M., Köktürk, F., & Kefeli, A. (2019). The protective and anti-inflammatory effect of methylene blue in corrosive esophageal burns: An experimental study. *Ulus Travma Acil Cerrahi Derg, 25*(4), 317-323. English. doi: 10.5505/tjtes.2018.58506

Seo, S., Choi, G., Lee, O., & Kang, H. (2022). Effect of methylene blue on experimental postoperative adhesion: A systematic review and meta-analysis. *PLoS One, 17*(5), e0268178. doi: 10.1371/journal.pone.0268178

Seong, D., & Kim, Y. (2015). Enhanced photodynamic therapy efficacy of methylene blue-loaded calcium phosphate nanoparticles. *J Photochem Photobiol B, 146*, 34-43. doi: 10.1016/j.jphotobiol.2015.02.022

Shareef, S., AlBarznji, M., Ahmed, S., Omer, T., Othman, Y., Amin, K., & Hama, R. (2024). Effectiveness of methylene blue as a local anesthetic and analgesic in perianal operations: A prospective double-blind randomized control trial. *Curr Probl Surg, 61*(8), 101521. doi: 10.1016/j.cpsurg.2024.101521

Shen, J., Jemec, G., Arendrup, M., & Saunte, D. (2020). Photodynamic therapy treatment of superficial fungal infections: A systematic review. *Photodiagnosis Photodyn Ther, 31*, 101774. doi: 10.1016/j.pdpdt.2020.101774

Shen, X., Dong, L., He, X., Zhao, C., Zhang, W., Li, X., & Lu, Y. (2020). Treatment of infected wounds with methylene blue photodynamic therapy: An effective and safe treatment method. *Photodiagnosis Photodyn Ther, 32*, 102051. doi: 10.1016/j.pdpdt.2020.102051

Shin, S., Kim, T., Wu, H., Choi, Y., & Kim, S. (2014). SIRT1 activation by methylene blue, a repurposed drug, leads to AMPK-mediated inhibition of steatosis and steatohepatitis. *Eur J Pharmacol, 727*, 115-24. doi: 10.1016/j.ejphar.2014.01.035

Shoelson, S., Lee, J., & Goldfine, A. (2006). Inflammation and insulin resistance. *J Clin Invest, 116*(8), 2308. doi: 10.1172/JCI29069E1. Erratum for: J Clin Invest. 116:1793.

Silva, A., Neves, C., Silva, E., Portela, T., Iunes, R., Cogliati, B., ... Silva, J. (2018). Effects of methylene blue-mediated photodynamic therapy on a mouse model of squamous cell carcinoma and normal skin. *Photodiagnosis Photodyn Ther, 23*, 154-164. doi: 10.1016/j.pdpdt.2018.06.012

Smith, E., Clark, M., Hardy, G., Kraan, D., Biondo, E., Gonzalez-Lima, F., ... Lee, H. (2017). Daily consumption of methylene blue reduces attentional deficits and dopamine reduction in a 6-OHDA model of Parkinson's disease. *Neuroscience, 359*, 8-16. doi: 10.1016/j.neuroscience.2017.07.001

Smith, E., Shaw, P., & De Vos, K. (2019). The role of mitochondria in amyotrophic lateral sclerosis. *Neurosci Lett, 710*, 132933. doi: 10.1016/j.neulet.2017.06.052

Souza, L., Souza, S., & Botelho, A. (2014). Distal and lateral toenail onychomycosis caused by Trichophyton rubrum: Treatment with photodynamic therapy based on methylene blue dye. *An Bras Dermatol, 89*(1), 184-6. doi: 10.1590/abd1806-4841.20142197

Sunela, K., & Bärlund, M. (2016). lfosfamidin aiheuttama enkefalopatia [Treatment and prevention of iphosphamide-induced encephalopathy]. *Duodecim,* *132*(4), 314-7. Finnish.

Sutherland, A., Faragher, I., & Frizelle, F. (2009). Intradermal injection of methylene blue for the treatment of refractory pruritus ani. *Colorectal Dis, 11*(3), 282-7. doi: 10.1111/j.1463-1318.2008.01587.x

Taldaev, A., Terekhov, R., Nikitin, I., Melnik, E., Kuzina, V., Klochko, M., ... Ramenskaya, G. (2023). Methylene blue in anticancer photodynamic therapy: Systematic review of preclinical studies. *Front Pharmacol, 14*, 1264961. doi: 10.3389/fphar.2023.1264961

Talley Watts, L., Long, J., Chemello, J., Van Koughnet, S., Fernandez, A., Huang, S., ... Duong, T. (2014). Methylene blue is neuroprotective against mild traumatic brain injury. *J Neurotrauma, 31*(11), 1063-71. doi: 10.1089/neu.2013.3193

Tariq, B., Simon, S., Pilz, W., Maxim, A., Kremer, B., & Baijens, L. (2021). Evaluating the safety of oral methylene blue during swallowing assessment: A systematic review. *Eur Arch Otorhinolaryngol, 278*(9), 3155-3169. doi: 10.1007/s00405-020-06509-3

Tardivo, J., Wainwright, M., & Baptista, M. (2015). Small scale trial of photodynamic treatment of onychomycosis in São Paulo. *J Photochem Photobiol B, 150*, 66-8. doi: 10.1016/j.jphotobiol.2015.03.015

Tardivo, J., Del Giglio, A., Paschoal, L., & Baptista, M. (2006). New photodynamic therapy protocol to treat AIDS-related Kaposi's sarcoma. *Photomed Laser Surg, 24*(4), 528-31. doi: 10.1089/pho.2006.24.528

Tardivo, J., Del Giglio, A., de Oliveira, C., Gabrielli, D., Junqueira, H., Tada, D., ... Baptista, M. (2005). Methylene blue in photodynamic therapy: From basic mechanisms to clinical applications. *Photodiagnosis Photodyn Ther, 2*(3), 175-91. doi: 10.1016/S1572-1000(05)00097-9

Torp, K., Modi, P., Pollard, E., & Simon, L. (2025). Pulse oximetry. [Updated 2023 Jul 30]. In: StatPearls [Internet]. Treasure Island (FL): StatPearls Publishing; Available from: https://www.ncbi.nlm.nih.gov/books/NBK470348/

Tucker, D., Lu, Y., & Zhang, Q. (2018). From mitochondrial function to neuroprotection-an emerging role for methylene blue. *Mol Neurobiol, 55*(6), 5137-5153. doi: 10.1007/s12035-017-0712-2

Turner, A., Duong, C., & Good, D. (2003). Methylene blue for the treatment and prophylaxis of ifosfamide-induced encephalopathy. *Clin Oncol (R Coll Radiol), 15*(7), 435-9. doi: 10.1016/s0936-6555(03)00114-6

Uhelski, M., Johns, M., Horrmann, A., Mohamed, S., Sohail, A., Khasabova, I., ... Banik, R. (2022). Adverse effects of methylene blue in peripheral neurons: An *in vitro* electrophysiology and cell culture study. *Mol Pain, 18*, 17448069221142523. doi: 10.1177/17448069221142523

Valenti, D., de Bari, L., De Filippis, B., Henrion-Caude, A., & Vacca, R. (2014). Mitochondrial dysfunction as a central actor in intellectual disability-related diseases: An overview of Down syndrome, autism, fragile X and Rett syndrome. *Neurosci Biobehav Rev, 46* Pt 2, 202-17. doi: 10.1016/j.neubiorev.2014.01.012

Waardenburg, S., de Meij, N., Brouwer, B., Van Zundert, J., & van Kuijk, S. (2022). Clinical important improvement of chronic pain patients in randomized controlled trials and the DATAPAIN cohort. *Pain Pract, 22*(3), 349-358. doi: 10.1111/papr.13089

Waingade, M., Medikeri, R., & Rathod, P. (2022). Effectiveness of methylene blue photosensitizers compared to that of corticosteroids in the management of oral lichen planus: A systematic review and meta-analysis. *J Dent Anesth Pain Med, 22*(3), 175-186. doi: 10.17245/jdapm.2022.22.3.175

Wang, C., & Wei, Y. (2017). Role of mitochondrial dysfunction and dysregulation of Ca^{2+} homeostasis in the pathophysiology of insulin resistance and type 2 diabetes. *J Biomed Sci, 24*(1), 70. doi: 10.1186/s12929-017-0375-3

Wang, J., Zhao, C., Kong, P., Bian, G., Sun, Z., Sun, Y., … Li, B. (2016). Methylene blue alleviates experimental autoimmune encephalomyelitis by modulating AMPK/SIRT1 signaling pathway and Th17/Treg immune response. *J Neuroimmunol, 299*, 45-52. doi: 10.1016/j.jneuroim.2016.08.014

Weissgerber, A. (2008) Methylene blue for refractory hypotension: a case report. *AANA J, 76*(4), 271-4

Wickramasinghe, D., Wickramasinghe, N., Samarasekera, N., & Warusavitarne, J. (2025). The effect of local infiltration of methylene blue on posthemorrhoidectomy pain: A systematic review and meta-analysis. *Curr Probl Surg, 67*, 101752. doi: 10.1016/j.cpsurg.2025.101752

Wiciński, M., Fajkiel-Madajczyk, A., Kurant, Z., Gryczka, K., Kurant, D., Szambelan, M., … Słupski, M. (2023). The use of cannabidiol in metabolic syndrome-An opportunity to improve the patient's health or much ado about nothing? *J Clin Med, 12*(14), 4620. doi: 10.3390/jcm12144620

Xiong, Z., O'Donovan, M., Sun, L., Choi, J., Ren, M., & Cao, K. (2017). Anti-aging potentials of methylene blue for human skin longevity. *Sci Rep, 7*(1), 2475. doi: 10.1038/s41598-017-02419-3

Xue, H., Thaivalappil, A., & Cao, K. (2021). The potentials of methylene blue as an anti-aging drug. *Cells, 10*(12), 3379. doi: 10.3390/cells10123379

Yang, L., Youngblood, H., Wu, C., & Zhang, Q. (2020). Mitochondria as a target for neuroprotection: Role of methylene blue and photobiomodulation. *Transl Neurodegener, 9*(1), 19. doi: 10.1186/s40035-020-00197-z

Yang, X., Lee, D., Kim, H., Park, B., Lim, C., & Bae, E. (2023). Cannabidiol inhibits IgE-mediated mast cell degranulation and anaphylaxis in mice. *Mol Nutr Food Res, 68*(3), e2300136. doi: 10.1002/mnfr.202300136

Yücel, Ö., Salabaş, E., Ermeç, B., & Kadıoğlu, A. (2017). The case report of Priapus and a modern approach to an ancient affliction. *Sex Med Rev, 5*(1):120-128. doi: 10.1016/j.sxmr.2016.08.003

Zakaria, S., Hoskin, T., & Degnim, A. (2008). Safety and technical success of methylene blue dye for lymphatic mapping in breast cancer. *Am J Surg, 196*(2), 228-33. doi: 10.1016/j.amjsurg.2007.08.060

Zhang, X., Rojas, J., & Gonzalez-Lima, F. (2006). Methylene blue prevents neurodegeneration caused by rotenone in the retina. *Neurotox Res, 9*(1), 47-57. doi: 10.1007/BF03033307

Zhang, Z., Liao, Y., Ai, B., & Liu, C. (2015). Methylene blue staining: A new technique for identifying intersegmental planes in anatomic segmentectomy. *Ann Thorac Surg, 99*(1), 238-42. doi: 10.1016/j.athoracsur.2014.07.071

Zhang, Z., Zhu, Z., Liu, H., Chen, J., Jin, C., & Zhang, X. (2025). A prospective, randomized, controlled trial of methylene blue injection for costal cartilage harvest postoperative analgesia. *Aesthet Surg J, 45*(2), NP65-NP70. doi: 10.1093/asj/sjae203

Zhao, N., Liang, P., Zhuo, X., Su, C., Zong, X., Guo, B., … Tie, X. (2018). After treatment with methylene blue is effective against delayed encephalopathy after acute carbon monoxide poisoning. *Basic Clin Pharmacol Toxicol, 122*(5), 470-480. doi: 10.1111/bcpt.12940

Zheng, J., & Li, Q. (2019). Methylene blue regulates inflammatory response in osteoarthritis by noncoding long chain RNA CILinc02. *J Cell Biochem, 120*(3), 3331-3338. doi: 10.1002/jcb.27602

Zheng, X., Ma, X., Li, T., Shi, W., & Zhang, Y. (2020). Effect of different drugs and drug combinations on killing stationary phase and biofilms recovered cells of Bartonella henselae in vitro. *BMC Microbiol, 20*(1), 87. doi: 10.1186/s12866-020-01777-9

Zoellner, L., Telch, M., Foa, E., Farach, F., McLean, C., Gallop, R., … Gonzalez-Lima, F. (2017). Enhancing extinction learning in posttraumatic stress disorder with brief daily imaginal exposure and methylene blue: A randomized controlled trial. *J Clin Psychiatry, 78*(7), e782-e789. doi: 10.4088/JCP.16m10936

Zou, J., Wang, X., Yang, Z., Yang, X., Wang, C., Sun, L., ... Nie, J. (2019) The application of methylene blue coloration technique in axillary lymph node dissection of breast cancer. *Transl Cancer Res, 8*(8), 2781-2790. doi: 10.21037/tcr.2019.10.42

Zuschlag, Z., Warren, M., & Schultz, S. (2018). Serotonin toxicity and urinary analgesics: A case report and systematic literature review of methylene blue-induced serotonin syndrome. *Psychosomatics, 59*(6), 539-546. doi: 10.1016/j.psym.2018.06.012

www.ingramcontent.com/pod-product-compliance
Lightning Source LLC
Chambersburg PA
CBHW051730020426
42333CB00014B/1244